'The second edition of this seminal work on Functional Analytic Psychotherapy (FAP) represents profound expansion and maturation of a groundbreaking approach. It builds on the original work by Robert Kohlenberg and his wife Mavis Tsai by adding a focus on the ACL model—living with Awareness, Courage, and Love— and linking their ideas to a process or principle based-approach more generally. An exciting and expanded group of excellent clinical authors elaborate on innovative ideas that enhance the therapist-client connection. It prepares the practitioner for a wide range of practical issues that will be confronted in creating deep, intimate, and transformative therapeutic relationships: from the therapeutic rationale to the ethics of relationship oriented work.

This updated volume is a testament to the enduring legacy of FAP and will serve as a vital resource for therapists seeking to integrate these principles into their practice. At once both gentle and inspiring, it invites both new and seasoned practitioners to cultivate a "sacred space" of trust and safety that allows growth and transformation. Beautifully and clearly written, it should be on every therapist's shelf who believes in the relevance of a functional analytic approach. I highly recommend it.'

Steven C. Hayes, PhD, *originator of Acceptance and Commitment Therapy (ACT)*

'This book is a must read for anyone who does FAP, is interested in learning FAP, or simply wants a way to harness the therapeutic relationship in their approach to clinical treatment. This second edition clearly positions FAP as a functional contextual therapy and recenters FAP based on behavioral principles. The interventions here will enhance the therapeutic relationship, lead to more intense connections, and help create more powerful clinical outcomes.'

Glenn Callaghan, PhD, *professor, San José State University*

'As a clinician who views the therapeutic relationship as the vehicle for behavior change, I am incredibly excited about *Functional Analytic Psychotherapy: Distinctive Features, 2nd Edition.* Knowing the authors' work and also knowing them personally, I can't think of a better group to convey the essential qualities of the relational process in psychotherapy and its potential impact. I recommend that every therapist read this book. Its capacity to support clinicians in creating a genuine therapy that clients will find life-changing can't be overstated.'

Robyn D. Walser, PhD, *licensed clinical psychologist and author of Heart of ACT, co-author of Mindful Couple: How Acceptance and Mindfulness Can Lead You to the Love You Want, Learning ACT II, The ACT Workbook for Anger, and ACT for Moral Injury*

'For years, data has shown us that the therapeutic relationship is perhaps the most powerful tool of change we have in psychotherapy. Functional Analytic Psychotherapy (FAP) therapists are the world experts on utilizing the therapeutic relationship with intention and precision, and I consider exposure to FAP to be invaluable to therapists of all traditions. In unpacking both the conceptual basis and clinical application of FAP in a series of well-written, pithy entries, this book is a perfect resource for clinicians who are new to FAP and as a reference for experienced hands to consult with questions about specific topics and applications. This excellent book should be on the shelf of every clinician who is interested in utilizing the power of the therapeutic relationship to full effect.'

Russell Kolts, PhD, *professor of psychology, Eastern Washington University, and author of* CFT Made Simple, Experiencing Compassion-Focused Therapy from the Inside Out, *and* The Anger Workbook

'The essence of functional analytic psychotherapy is simply to understand the functions of our "outputs". Those outputs may be speech acts, actual behaviors, emotion expressions, or motive pursuits. FAP rarely takes things at face value but helps us explore and understand the function (reasons and hopes) of our ways of processing and generating responses. These can arise from both conscious and non-conscious processing. The therapist also helps us to explore other ways goals can be achieved. The second edition of this book is a masterful overview of FAP in various forms of interaction including the therapeutic relationship. It is well written, with many excellent clinical examples and a source of therapeutic wisdoms compassionately delivered that will be of great value to therapists whatever their preferred model. It's FAB!'

Paul Gilbert, PhD, OBE, *author of* Compassion Focused Therapy *and* The Compassionate Mind

'In the 1980s, as a student of behaviorism and devoted follower of B. F. Skinner, I attended a tiny regional conference in Victoria, British Columbia. There, I met Bob Kohlenberg. As the only undergraduate—and a thirty-something who was less than three years out of drug rehab—I felt nervous and out of place, yet I was deeply passionate about the subject. At a dinner party after the conference, Bob treated me with tremendous respect as he walked me through a behavioral interpretation of the interpersonal exchange in psychodynamic psychotherapy.

Three years later, Bob and Mavis Tsai published the first book on Functional Analytic Psychotherapy (FAP), a guide for creating intense and curative therapeutic relationships. That conversation, which implicitly affirmed the importance of my own inner world, has resonated with me throughout my career and informed my own therapy and supervision. Unlike the almost exclusively client-facing approaches of Cognitive Behavioral Therapy (CBT), FAP addresses the complexities that emerge within therapists as they practice. FAP views the therapist's inner world not as a nuisance to be managed, but as a crucial stream of data. The therapist's inner world serves as a guide for navigating the therapeutic alliance and is our closest source of insight into the interpersonal challenges faced by our clients.

I encourage serious therapists, who seek more than psycho-therapy cookbooks, to explore the newly revised *Functional Analytic Psychotherapy: Distinctive Features*. This book invites readers into a deeper exploration of this essential subject matter.'

Kelly Wilson, PhD, *professor emeritus, University of Mississippi, and founder of OneLife, LLC*

'*Functional Analytic Psychotherapy: Distinctive Features* offers an accessible and enjoyable overview of what sets FAP apart, conceptually and practically. This text isn't just about making converts, however. By offering the reader a chance to explore the therapeutic relationship from the behaviorist perspective on which FAP is based, the authors invite and empower the reader to integrate FAP into their existing practices. This revised edition will be especially useful for anyone seeking to nurture deep, authentic relationships with clients even across disparities in power, privilege, and positionality.'

Emily K. Sandoz, BCBA, PhD, *Louisiana Contextual Science Research Group, UL Lafayette, and Camélia House Counseling*

Functional Analytic Psychotherapy

Following in the steps of the first edition, *Functional Analytic Psychotherapy: Distinctive Features, 2nd Edition*, provides a history, context, and building blocks for a behavior therapist to incorporate Functional Analytic Psychotherapy (FAP) into their work.

This new volume updates material based upon research that has occurred since the first edition, as well as philosophical and theoretical shifts in behavior therapy, such as an emphasis on FAP as a process-based therapy. Each FAP principle is presented in terms of its intended purpose and is clearly linked to the underlying theory, providing clinicians with a straightforward guide for when and how to apply each technique. Practical tips have been added to aid in case conceptualization and the integration of a FAP framework into other process-based, behavioral conceptualizations. The added breadth and depth also emphasize FAP's unique role in meeting the needs of diverse and marginalized people and applying FAP across diverse settings.

This book will be an important read for any student, trainee, or CBT practitioner.

Amanda Muñoz-Martínez is a clinical psychologist, certified FAP trainer, and an associate professor at the Universidad de Los Andes, Colombia.

Matthew D. Skinta is an associate professor of psychology and affiliated faculty of women and gender studies at Roosevelt University.

Sarah Sullivan-Singh is a psychologist, clinical instructor in the psychology department of the University of Washington, and a certified FAP trainer who specializes in working with adults experiencing health-related adversity.

Barbara Kohlenberg is a professor at the University of Nevada Reno School of Medicine and is a clinical psychologist interested in contextual behavioral science, particularly FAP and Acceptance and Commitment Therapy (ACT).

Mavis Tsai is a senior research scientist at the University of Washington and co-creator of FAP.

CBT Distinctive Features

Series Editor: Windy Dryden

Cognitive behaviour therapy (CBT) occupies a central position in the move towards evidence-based practice and is frequently used in the clinical environment. Yet there is no one universal approach to CBT and clinicians speak of first-, second-, and even third-wave approaches.

This series provides straightforward, accessible guides to a number of CBT methods, clarifying the distinctive features of each approach. The series editor, Windy Dryden successfully brings together experts from each discipline to summarise the 30 main aspects of their approach divided into theoretical and practical features.

The CBT Distinctive Features Series will be essential reading for psychotherapists, counsellors, and psychologists of all orientations who want to learn more about the range of new and developing cognitive behaviour approaches.

Recent titles in the series:

For further information about this series please visit
www.routledge.com/CBT-Distinctive-Features/book-series/DFS

Functional Analytic Psychotherapy

Distinctive Features

2nd Edition

Amanda Muñoz-Martínez, Matthew D. Skinta, Sarah Sullivan-Singh, Barbara Kohlenberg, and Mavis Tsai

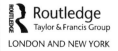

Routledge
Taylor & Francis Group

LONDON AND NEW YORK

Second edition published 2025
by Routledge
4 Park Square, Milton Park, Abingdon, Oxon, OX14 4RN

and by Routledge
605 Third Avenue, New York, NY 10158

Routledge is an imprint of the Taylor & Francis Group, an informa business

First edition published by Routledge 2012

British Library Cataloguing-in-Publication Data
A catalogue record for this book is available from the British Library

Library of Congress Cataloging-in-Publication Data
Names: Muñoz-Martínez, Amanda, author. | Tsai, Mavis, author.
Title: Functional analytic psychotherapy: distinctive features / Amanda Muñoz-Martínez, Matthew D. Skinta, Sarah Sullivan-Singh, Barbara Kohlenberg, Mavis Tsai.
Description: Second edition. | New York: Routledge, 2024. | Series: CBT distinctive features series | Revised edition of: Functional analytic psychotherapy / Mavis Tsai ... [et al.]. Hove, East Sussex; New York: Routledge, 2012. | Includes bibliographical references and index.
Identifiers: LCCN 2024026153 | ISBN 9781032694856 (hardback) | ISBN 9781032687179 (paperback) | ISBN 9781032694832 (ebook)
Subjects: LCSH: Behavior therapy. | Psychoanalysis.
Classification: LCC RC489.B4 F86 2024 | DDC 616.89/142--dc23/eng/20240909
LC record available at https://lccn.loc.gov/2024026153

ISBN: 9781032694856 (hbk)
ISBN: 9781032687179 (pbk)
ISBN: 9781032694832 (ebk)

DOI: 10.4324/9781032694832

Typeset in Times New Roman
by Deanta Global Publishing Services, Chennai, India

To my Dad, Alejandro, I feel the absence of your love every day. To Yors, you continue teaching me what love takes and what love makes. To my Mom, Brother, and Sister-cousin, you are my natural reinforcers, purely unconditional.
– AMM

For my husband, Barthélémy, who pushes me to always take risks; and for the wonderful friends who naturally reinforce my bids for a life filled with vulnerability and intimacy.
– MDS

For Mom, Dad, and Rachel, who first taught me the dance of love; and for Virtaj, the biggest and most loving evoke I could ever desire.
– SSS

For my parents, Bob Kohlenberg and Joan Giacomini, who gave me the blueprint for love, and to my children, who have indeed shown me the varied landscapes of love.
– BK

To Bob, whose spirit and love continue to guide and inspire every step I take.
– MT

Contents

About the authors

Amanda Muñoz-Martínez is a clinical psychologist and certified FAP trainer. She is an associate professor at the Universidad de Los Andes, Colombia, pioneering investigations in Contextual Behavioral Science therapies, such as FAP, and social connection in the Latin American population. She has a clinical practice and provides ongoing training and supervision in FAP.

Matthew D. Skinta is an associate professor of psychology and affiliated faculty of women and gender studies at Roosevelt University, a peer-reviewed Acceptance and Commitment Therapy (ACT) trainer, certified FAP trainer, and Compassion Cultivation Training teacher. He is a Fellow of the Association for Contextual Behavioral Science, the Association for Behavioral and Cognitive Therapies, and the American Psychological Association (Divisions 44 and 52).

Sarah Sullivan-Singh is a psychologist and certified FAP trainer who specializes in working with adults experiencing health-related adversity. In addition to providing psychotherapy, supervision, and consultation services, she co-leads The Seattle Clinic, a collaborative of independent mental health practitioners, and facilitates FAP workshops.

Barbara Kohlenberg is a clinical psychologist interested in contextual behavioral science, particularly in FAP and ACT. Barbara teaches and consults with psychiatry residents who are learning psychotherapy and works with family medicine residents who are interested in brief mental health interventions in a primary care setting. Barbara presents workshops in FAP and provides direct patient care.

Mavis Tsai co-created FAP with Robert Kohlenberg, PhD, ABPP. A senior research scientist at the University of Washington, she is a recipient of Washington State's Distinguished Psychologist Award and is a Fellow of the Association for Contextual Behavioral Science. She founded the nonprofit Awareness, Courage & Love Global Project to bring FAP to the general public.

Preface

Functional Analytic Psychotherapy (FAP) is a behavioral approach to psychotherapy based on empirically supported principles that harness the power of the therapeutic relationship and maximize the genuineness, intensity, compassion, and effectiveness of the therapist. FAP therapists view each client as a microculture with complex life stories of joy and anguish, dreams and hopes, passions and vulnerabilities, and unique gifts and abilities, carrying deeply rooted cultural, social, and generational experiences in their reinforcement histories.

The importance of the therapeutic relationship is not unique to FAP. This emphasis is asserted in all Cognitive-Behavioral Therapy (CBT) approaches, although none elevate it to the central role it has in FAP. The difficulty is that nearly everyone means something different by the concept of the therapeutic relationship, and it has a history of nuances and definitions that date back to Sigmund Freud. Given these complexities and often deeply held preconceptions, our challenge is to present the FAP viewpoint briefly and yet clearly distinguish it from existing notions. Thus, this book distills the core principles, techniques, and vision of FAP into 30 short chapters that emphasize its power as a precise behavioral theory leading to flexible, compassionate, intimate, and powerful therapeutic relationships that supercharge any CBT treatment. The chapters are written to maximize clarity and understanding for all readers, including those without a behavioral background, those who wish to add FAP techniques to their ongoing work, and those already familiar with FAP wishing to expand their expertise.

This book presents behavioral theory and FAP techniques in terms that clarify their purpose and show how they can lead to deep, intense therapeutic relationships with pragmatic examples demonstrating their utility for both simple and complex cases. Part I of this volume delves into the historical roots and evolution of FAP as a principle-based therapy. We explore FAP's foundation in understanding the function of behaviors and the pivotal role of verbal behavior in understanding therapeutic interactions. Central to FAP is the conception of the therapeutic relationship as a genuine relationship, underpinned by the central role of natural reinforcement as the key to building meaningful relations and connections. For this endeavor, therapists are required to identify Clinically Relevant Behaviors (CRBs) that categorize clients' in-session behaviors. We examine how FAP targets interpersonal repertoires, emphasizing the significance of emotions, feelings, and the development and support of the self within the therapeutic process. Furthermore, we address the awareness, courage, and love (ACL) model of intimacy in FAP, as well as the importance of vulnerability in context. Ethical considerations, alongside the imperative discussion of diversity, privilege, power, and justice, are highlighted to underscore FAP's commitment to addressing complex social dynamics within therapy. Through this comprehensive overview, therapists are invited to appreciate FAP's nuanced approach to enriching the therapist-client relationship and fostering profound personal growth and connection.

Part II provides a step-by-step guide to the application of FAP techniques and rules, starting with the importance of creating a sacred space for trust and safety, a foundational aspect to build up a curative and intense therapeutic relationship. This section delves into functional analysis and case conceptualization, equipping practitioners with the tools to identify the functions of the client's behavior within and outside of the session. FAP rules are presented in terms of their intended function, so each therapeutic procedure is clearly linked to the underlying theory, providing clinicians with not just a description of the technique but also a simple guide for when and how to use each one. We also discuss some fundamentals in the training and supervision of therapists. Finally, we introduce some special areas of interest for FAP therapists, such as grief, interventions in health settings, and integration with other therapies.

Given the potential importance of the therapeutic relationship to help therapists of any theoretical approach achieve therapeutic goals, this book contains concrete suggestions about how to intensify here-and-now therapeutic interactions. Consistent with an integrationist emphasis, specific guidelines are given so that therapists can use FAP concepts along with existing CBT treatments to deal with a wide range of significant clinical issues such as intimacy, problems of the self, and attachment.

In recent years, empirically based treatments have sparked increased interest in understanding the mechanisms underlying their results, as well as in producing changes that enhance diverse populations' well-being. FAP has exponentially grown in this respect, consolidating a mature therapeutic approach deeply rooted in principles aimed at promoting individuals' interpersonal functioning and social connection, two crucial aspects for enhancing people's quality of life. Recent research suggests that FAP's mechanism of change is valid and can lead to significant changes in clients. With more research and training planned over the coming years, an explosion of interest in FAP is anticipated as these results become more widely known. Regardless of your orientation or where you are in your journey as a psychotherapist, we hope the ideas and information contained in this book will inspire you intellectually and facilitate the development of therapeutic relationships that are extraordinary and meaningful.

Amanda Muñoz-Martínez
Matthew D. Skinta
Sarah Sullivan-Singh
Barbara Kohlenberg
Mavis Tsai

Acknowledgments

Amanda Muñoz-Martínez:

I am profoundly grateful to my co-authors Mathew, Sarah, Barbara, and Mavis for their dedication and brilliant contributions. Especially, Mavis, thank you for inviting this diverse group of FAPers to contribute to an already fantastic book. The insights and collaborative spirit of this team enriched our work immensely, making this journey not just educational but truly reinforcing. I believe we have shaped a book full of renewed, reconciled, and vibrant ideas for implementing FAP.

I thank my mentors, Mónica Novoa and Bill Follette. Mónica introduced me to FAP and instilled in me the belief that I would find a magical place where behavioral principles and the therapeutic relationship reconcile. Bill guided me toward discovering the heart of FAP; my therapeutic practice and research approach were transformed by his unparalleled wisdom.

I am incredibly thankful to my students and trainees for their support and trust in my guidance. Your curiosity, enthusiasm, and commitment to learning have not only supported me but have also been a constant source of inspiration. Without you, my ideas and teachings would be nothing. Your belief in our shared path has been a driving force in our collective pursuit of knowledge and growth.

To my clients, your trust has shown me the beauty of connection and the privilege of accompanying your journeys. I thank my loved ones, who have enriched my life with profound relationships and courageously navigated life's challenges with me. Your influence is immeasurable, and I am eternally grateful for your companionship and support in all facets of my life.

Lastly, I thank FAP itself for transforming my professional and personal life. FAP has helped me to become a better person who is ongoingly growing.

Matthew D. Skinta:

I deeply appreciate and value the vision, brilliance, and clinical acumen of my co-authors, Amanda, Sarah, Barbara, and Mavis, and feel so privileged to be included in this work. FAP as both a therapy and FAP therapists as a community benefit from the ways that it is enacted and practiced in the world, shaped and embodied through increasingly diverse sets of our learning histories and varied stimulus values in the room. I thank Beth Wildman, my professor at Kent State University, who first suggested I might enjoy the first book on FAP, setting me on this journey.

I have had a number of amazing students, trainees, and supervisees over the years who have inspired me with their own innovations and exploration of creating sacred, intimate spaces in the therapy room. My clients in my years of private practice have taught me more than I could have imagined about the power of extending a loving invitation to grow, and seeing the direction they take it when the relationship and their behaviors feel tended to and cared about. My current students mirror and reflect back to me the excitement I felt, and the hunger, for an approach deeply grounded in the science of learning theory while simultaneously being heartfelt, meaningful, and relational.

Finally, I offer the deepest thanks and gratitude to Mavis Tsai and Bob Kohlenberg for creating this beautiful gift to the world that continues to enrich my life.

Sarah Sullivan-Singh:
What a privilege it has been to muse and write about FAP with my wise and astute co-authors, Amanda, Matthew, Barbara, and Mavis! No matter how many times I approach the principles of FAP, I continue encountering new facets of this contextual behavioral gem that Mavis and Bob originally unearthed. I am immensely grateful for the relationships with mentors, colleagues, trainees, clients, friends, and family members alike that offer valiant invitations to take courageous risks, genuine reinforcement of my 2s, and compassionate acceptance of me, right along with my 1s.

Special thanks to (in order of appearance): Katie Paul, my irreplaceable, lifelong friend, whose abiding presence defines home to me and functions as a basecamp for all my quests; Tom Doelger, my sage English teacher, who forgave my inappropriate use of commas, illuminated the humanity in every story, and heard my voice before I could; Annette Stanton, my unwavering dissertation advisor, who stayed in the boat with me even when I lost my compass (and the oars); Betina Yanez, my brilliant lab-, room-, and life-mate, whose capacity for unconditional love has yet to stop expanding my heart; Kauser Ahmed, my percipient supervisor, who taught me to meet my clients and their mysteries with curiosity and reverence; Mary Loudon, my cardinal passage into FAP, whose courageous example showed me how to bring my essential self into the room as an authentic healing channel—and who keeps inviting my whole self to unfurl along with hers; and Julia Hitch, my protean colleague and comrade, whose affectionate and attuned persistence fortifies my spirit and emboldens me to try evoking one more time. Your love is in all my words that follow.

Barbara Kohlenberg:

My father, Bob Kohlenberg, reflected that it delighted him to notice that when his children learned to talk, the few words they each had blossomed into many, and then they were talking to each other and to everyone. I know that he would be moved and delighted to see that the ideas and principles articulated in FAP together with Mavis have spread throughout the world and have impacted so many lives. I imagine the two of them, in the early days, intensely working out the articulation of FAP, talking about it, writing about it, the first book, involving their students and their professional communities, and now people around the world are talking about FAP and/or have had their lives changed because of it. No higher honor for my father.

My brilliant and tender co-authors, Matthew, Amanda, and Sarah, honor his memory so deeply by diving deeply into FAP and making it their own. My clients, over the years, who have taught me and honored me by sharing their hearts with me, and who hold both my mistakes and my steadfast commitment to their well-being in such a loving way. And of course, to Mavis Tsai, who is the sine qua non of this volume and of this work, in every way. Thank all of you for showing that FAP is about what we do, that love is behavior, and that good things happen when both heart and science walk together.

Mavis Tsai:

In the profound absence of Bob Kohlenberg, my partner in life and work for an unforgettable span of 43 years, I am enveloped in a tapestry of emotions that traverse the essence of love, loss, legacy, and the unyielding power of human connection. His groundbreaking ideas continue to resonate through the hearts and minds of countless individuals, perpetuating a legacy that transcends the bounds of time. It is in this spirit that I extend my deepest appreciation to Amanda, Matthew, Sarah, and Barbara—my remarkable team of co-authors. Their brilliance and dedication have been instrumental in co-writing this edition.

Jonathan Kanter, Gareth Holman, and Mary Plummer Loudon, my esteemed co-authors of the first edition, alongside Bob, crafted a foundational masterpiece that intertwined intellect and heart, setting a magnificent foundation for this current work.

In the aftermath of Bob's passing, Barbara Kohlenberg, Bob's cherished daughter, has been my companion through the shadowed valleys of grief. Valerie Freilich, my dearest friend, has been a pillar of support, walking with me through the darkness and back into the light, helping me find my way in life without Bob.

Bob wholeheartedly supported the formation of my nonprofit organization, the Awareness, Courage & Love (ACL) Global Project, which brings FAP principles to the general public. In my time of grief, I've been uplifted by the love and inspiration of my beloved FAP and ACL colleagues from around the world. Ben Spaloss, a Gen Z leader who is co-writing a book on ACL with me, embodies the joy and promise of what lies ahead.

My heart is filled with immeasurable gratitude for all my students, trainees, and clients, both past and present. They are the architects of my spirit and a wellspring for my dedication to FAP. They each hold a unique and irreplaceable space in my heart.

As we turn the pages of this second edition, let us honor the past, embrace the present, and look forward to a future bright with promise and potential. Together, we continue the journey, guided by awareness, driven by courage, inspired by love, and united by the transformative power of FAP.

Part I

THE DISTINCTIVE THEORETICAL FEATURES OF FAP

This section aims to introduce the foundational components of FAP, including its historical roots, theoretical underpinnings, and key concepts for implementation. It also covers elements from the professional areas of interest within the FAP community, such as ethics and diversity.

DOI: 10.4324/9781032694832-1

The historical roots of Functional Analytic Psychotherapy

Behaviorism is the theoretical scientific basis upon which Functional Analytic Psychotherapy (FAP) rests. Behaviorism has the advantages of a strong, laboratory empirical base, operationally defined concepts, and precise language. These advantages establish a theory, that in turn, produces effective techniques that can be taught precisely to others. The result of this endeavor is Functional Analytic Psychotherapy, an intervention that can be used as a stand-alone therapy or be integrated and bring intensity and "magic" to any other therapeutic approach.

FAP is not the first to use behavioral concepts to define an exceptionally effective but somewhat mysterious and unteachable clinical treatment. C. B. Ferster (1967a), an early behaviorist, studied an extremely talented therapist who obtained amazing results in her treatment of autistic children. Others who tried to emulate her were not effective. Her approach was purely intuitive, and she could not coherently describe why she did what she did. Dr Ferster intensively observed her work over a long period. He used behavioral concepts to describe what she did, as well as to account for her amazing effects. Needless to say, this process led to an understandable, non-mysterious, and, most important, teachable treatment that was the forerunner of today's treatment practices for severely disturbed children.

C. B. Ferster (1979) also proposed several applications of behavioral principles for understanding and modifying problematic behaviors of verbally able clients in psychotherapy. He described the importance of creating a naturally reinforcing environment at the beginning of therapy so that therapists can establish themselves as sources of reinforcement. He also would advise therapists to take advantage of the therapeutic setting to reinforce clients' behaviors as they occurred instead of focusing on verbal descriptions of clients' intended actions outside of the session. In other words, C. B. Ferster (1979) set a framework in which

DOI: 10.4324/9781032694832-2

direct contingencies as described in FAP would be the most valuable tools to promote exceptional therapeutic outcomes.

The origin of Functional Analytic Psychotherapy (FAP) is associated with most practicing therapists reporting surprising and remarkable findings that go beyond standard treatment outcomes. Even when following a manual and using standardized procedures, some of our clients achieve gains that go far beyond the intended goal of symptom alleviation or of obtaining remission from a DSM (Diagnostic and Statistical Manual of Mental Disorders IV, American Psychiatric Association, 2000) defined disorder. We will refer to these phenomena as "exceptionally good outcomes." Most of us, especially in this era of empirically supported treatments, do help most of our clients. The phenomena we are talking about, however, go beyond this usual "good" outcome or what has been called "specific factors." Although most patients are helped, needless to say, the obverse side of these exceptionally good outcomes is those clients for whom the same methods that seem to help others are mysteriously unsuccessful. Those differences have been usually attributed to so-called "unspecific factors" such as therapeutic alliance. There is something special in the therapist-client relationship. The therapist-client relationship frequently is invoked to explain differential outcomes (e.g., Horvath, 2001); however, exactly how and why the therapeutic relationship affects outcomes and what the therapist can do to influence this relationship in order to obtain these exceptional outcomes are less well specified. For this reason, and for want of a better word, we will temporarily refer to this difficult-to-describe quality as "magic" in the therapy room.

In our experience and in interviewing colleagues about what was different about these exceptional cases, one commonality emerged that captured these exceptional cases. Intensity, personal involvement, and frequent moment-to-moment therapist-client exchanges made these clients and the therapy experiences unforgettable. If you are concerned that our use of the term "magic" means we believe there is a mysterious, new age, perhaps paranormal phenomenon that therapists must learn to harness, nothing could be farther from the truth. Further, we do not believe that master therapists have the magic spark and that the rest of us are doomed to do "good" but not "exceptional" work. Instead, our task is to understand what kinds of therapist actions (interventions) bring about the phenomena that seem magical. Our recommendations must be well-specified, easy to understand, and easily teachable to others.

Another advantage of using behaviorism to explain why and how exceptional outcomes are obtained is that it does not suffer from the downfall of other similar attempts to capture the essential elements of why some therapists do better than others. Most notably, there is a long-standing tradition in our field of studying "master therapists," those who routinely help clients achieve exceptionally good outcomes (Shapiro, 1987). The process entails studying the superstar therapist, observing what they do, and then teaching others to emulate it. The downfall, according to Shapiro, is that imitating the exact behaviors of a successful therapist does not take into account that what works for one therapist may not work for another. In contrast, the process used by Ferster, described above, developed general abstract principles that accommodated contextual differences between therapists and clients (i.e., used functional analysis as discussed later in this book) and avoided the "one size fits all" problem.

Similarly, FAP is not a set of specific procedures. Instead, it is a set of general principles based on behaviorism. It is important to emphasize that in order to implement FAP you do not have to be a behaviorist. However, FAP effects can be boosted by your knowledge of those principles as you would be able to identify which of your behaviors as a therapist might be more successful in modifying a particular problem using specific procedures under specific circumstances.

The road map of FAP leads to and explores the core of psychotherapy, the therapeutic relationship. Grounded in behavioral principles, FAP adeptly handles a broad spectrum of behavioral issues, especially those not covered by standard diagnostic criteria like the DSM or those without established treatments, yet significantly impacts well-being (Kanter et al., 2010). FAP's positive effects on clients' social interactions underscore FAP's transformative potential in clinical practice (Singh & O'Brien, 2018).

2

FAP as a principle-based therapy

Many practitioners in clinical psychology, particularly in CBT, have traditionally adopted Empirically Based Treatments (EBT) in their practice. However, recent scrutiny of EBT foundations has raised questions about their utility beyond efficacy in controlled environments. This examination encompasses their mechanisms of change, practical application, connection to basic science, applicability in diverse and natural contexts, and their impact on well-being beyond symptom reduction (Tolin et al., 2015). Consequently, practitioners and researchers are starting to transform their practices and challenge the system that identifies an intervention as empirically based.

In response to calls for transformation in clinical science, contextual behavioral therapies are shifting their focus toward investigating processes rather than diagnosis. These therapies define processes as "a set of theory-based, dynamic, progressive, and multilevel changes that occur in predictable empirically established sequences oriented toward the desirable outcomes" (Hayes & Hoffman, 2019, p. 38). Hayes and Hoffman (2019) have proposed developing a research agenda that shifts clinical science from a nomothetic-based to an idiographic-oriented approach. By adopting Process-Based Treatments (PBT), they argue that, we can build a coordinated agenda in clinical science that overcomes the barriers imposed by traditional therapeutic models, which have been redundant, context-insensitive, and unscalable. They suggest that PBT should embrace evolutionary science as the framework for explaining psychological problems and interventions through the dynamics of three key principles: selection, retention, and variation, and its influence across different processes (affective, cognitive, attentional, self, motivation, overt behavior; Sanford et al., 2022; Hayes et al., 2020).

While some contextual therapies, such as Acceptance and Commitment Therapy (ACT), have urgently responded to this call, FAP has sounded a more subtle alarm. For some researchers, FAP

DOI: 10.4324/9781032694832-3

naturally suits PBT characteristics as an idiographic, contextually sensitive, functional, and principle-rooted intervention (Maitland, 2024). Originating as a *principle-based therapy*, FAP has acted in line with behavioral principles based on basic science and grounded in theory, particularly the principle of *reinforcement* (Kohlenberg & Tsai, 1991). *Reinforcement* principle describes the probability that after a given consequence is presented the chances of occurrence of the behavior increase in the future, a behavioral principle with extensive evidence and applicability (Williams, 1983). Other principles such as discrimination (the ability to differentiate between stimuli), extinction (behavior reduction due to the discontinuation of reinforcement), generalization (the emission of behavior in situations different from where it was learned), and punishment (behavior reduction as a result of withdrawing or providing a stimulus) explain the therapeutic outcomes of FAP. In order to move these mechanisms, FAP therapists utilize therapeutic, widely tested behavior analytic procedures such as shaping, modeling, and differentially reinforcing, among others (Muñoz-Martínez et al., 2022).

FAP researchers faced challenges in empirically testing how reinforcement operates in therapy sessions, as this requires examining the dynamics between therapists and clients to bridge the gap in treatment-outcome research. Despite delays in meeting the earlier EBT criteria set by Chambless and Hollon (1998), FAP's idiographic and functional stance on clients' behaviors and its grounding in basic science principles align well with more recent EBT criteria (Tolin et al., 2015). This book invites readers to adopt a principle-based intervention perspective, focusing on how well-tested principles can help change contingencies in the therapy room. It encourages confidence in basic science's ability to explain treatment outcomes. By wearing the "glasses" of a principle-based approach, readers can gain a deeper understanding of how FAP's strategies and interventions work to facilitate multi-level therapeutic change, as well as embracing therapists' capacity as change-makers in the therapy room.

3

What's the function?

Every client enters a therapy session with a lifetime of history accompanying them. FAP therapists have the good fortune of being able to be curious about the unique meaning and function of any and all behavior that enters the session. The client who has not done their homework, or has done their homework very meticulously, the client who brings a gift of cookies, the client who writes a poem for the therapist, the client who brings expensive concert tickets to the therapist, the client who arrives an hour early, for every session, the client who is frequently late. How do you, as a therapist, respond?

Many cognitive-behavioral and other therapies have standard answers to these behaviors. Typically, one might react with concern for forgotten or incomplete homework and with genuine pleasure for completed, meticulous homework. Gifts of cookies or a poem might be accepted warmly. The expensive concert tickets might evoke concern from the therapist and likely a kind reminder about boundaries and office policy about not accepting gifts. We might appreciate a client who arrives early, feeling that they must value therapy a great deal. We might want to discontinue treatment for a client who is chronically late or interpret the behavior as a problem. In FAP, however, we would want to look at these more deeply and contextually, not respond only based on the form of the behavior. We would want to know the function of these behaviors. Ways to appreciate function generally involve these kinds of questions: (a) What are the contexts that evoke the behavior? and (b) What are the consequences that make it more or less likely? With respect to homework being done or not done, knowing what is usually true for the client is meaningful. Do they have a history of never doing homework, do they always do it, are there distractions that interfere with doing it? And with respect to consequences, we may explore how therapists, teachers, or other authority figures have punished or rewarded homework completion in the past. Has the client been hurt

DOI: 10.4324/9781032694832-4

due to not doing homework well enough or is there worried that doing homework well might mean care will be withdrawn because the client is functioning so well with their homework. Has the client had therapists who assign homework and then not ask about it?

With respect to client gifts of cookies, a poem, an expensive concert ticket, thinking about contexts that surround giving, would help to understand the function. Is the gift about thanks for feeling very helped, is it a prelude to asking for a favor, is it an avoidance of expressing verbally deep feelings for the therapist, might it be related to previous trauma by a health care practitioner (such as racial trauma) and wanting to be sure to be liked and not harmed. Did the client come from a family where gifts were rare and painful to give or receive or were gifts culturally accepted and plentiful. The client who is very early to each session, one might wonder about histories of being late, about the meaning of time alone in the waiting room. The client who is late, is this harmful to the relationship or might it be an improvement, coming instead of canceling, or perhaps being late functions to express anger that might be useful to note and to talk about in session.

An analysis of the context and consequences allows for considering many possibilities when understanding the function of behavior. Is the client someone who struggles with being overly concerned with pleasing others and is trying out not doing homework to see how the therapist will respond? In this case, not doing homework could be an improvement, a CRB2. Or is the client avoiding doing homework because they are anxious that it is not good enough, this could be a CRB1 (see Chapter 7 for a throughout definition of CRBs). It also could be the case that the client had car trouble and a sick child and was distracted by other life demands, so, not doing the homework would not be clinically relevant.

Similarly, a client who is very shy and struggles to demonstrate appreciation and brings the therapist a gift may be showing improvement in expression of caring, a CRB2. A client who wants something from the therapist, such as an extended work excuse and the therapist does not agree with this, and the client attempts to bribe the therapist with a gift, would be a CRB1. Giving a gift related to "please don't hurt me," rather than talking about fears based on past relationships may be an opportunity to talk deeply about the trauma history and the gift may be more about avoidance, which would be a CRB1. An expensive gift, while unlikely to ever be acceptable to accept, would be an opportunity to explore the function of the gift with the therapist, and the history of giving expensive gifts, is the client hoping to incur favor, is the client hoping to buy love due to a history of not being cared about for their deeper qualities.

FAP adds to what many therapies do when trying to interpret client behavior. The FAP analysis adds structure to this exploration by focusing on behavioral function as the key to understanding the behavior and to link therapist responses to the behavioral functions identified.

All clinically relevant behavior (CRB) in FAP is to be explored and understood functionally in this way. What is the function of tears, anger, requests, focus, or avoidance of certain topics in session? Out of session, what is the function of these same kinds of behaviors? Asking "what is the function" is an essential question for a FAP therapist, it is fundamental to FAP's Rule 1 (Watch for CRB's Clinically Relevant Behaviors; see Chapter 20). Asking "what is the function?" takes in the history and humanity of each of our clients and encourages emotionally intimate connections in the therapeutic interaction.

4

Verbal behavior: The roots of FAP interactions

If a man says to his therapist, "As a depressed person, I often have a hard time describing my feelings to my friends," what does he mean? Should this be interpreted as an accurate description of his own behavior that he has observed and noted, or have the responses of other people around him slowly shaped his responses based on what leads to attention, affection, or desired care from others?

While the content of a client's speech might be meaningful, it is important to consider what the function of a given type of speech serves. Beyond the common functions of our social behaviors, such as feelings of connection, warmth, attention, or touch, our means of expression and use of words are the result of thousands of small interactions where the responses of others shape how we express ourselves.

One question typically avoided by the behavior therapist is the question: "Why?" This is because across many cultures, the norms of verbal behavior suggest that one should be aware of the causes of one's own behavior, willing to disclose them, and that they should make a certain sense to the listener. Other people might respond positively to a good explanation in response to "Why?" or respond with discomfort or distance themselves from those unable to answer such questions. The famed behaviorist B. F. Skinner referred to the stories evoked by the question "Why?" as explanatory fictions. We are constantly, in various situations and across contexts, encouraged to have answers or explain our behavior. It would be a mistake to assume that the stories we have developed or learned to tell are accurate descriptions of our behavior and its causes. Our behavior and our habits of storytelling are, after all, different types of behavior than accurately reporting recent events (Hineline, 1983).

Skinner encourages the behavior therapist to think in terms of function and developed a broad vocabulary for categorizing language into

DOI: 10.4324/9781032694832-5

its functional class. One helpful term used to understand verbal behavior, for instance, is the *tact*. Tacting, derived from the word "contact" by Skinner, refers to verbal behavior that attaches a label or description to an experience (private or public) that then is shaped by the reinforcing or punishing behavior of others. For example, a child noting that an apple is "red" is tacting, and labeling this perceived color likely leads to excitement or responsiveness from adults if this is a new and exciting behavior. One is similarly tacting when describing private event, such as hunger, sadness, or joy (Skinner, 1957). Another helpful term to be aware of is the *mand*, derived from words such as "demand" or "command." The function of a mand is defined by a consequence that typically follows. For example, it would be a mand to ask, "May I have a glass of water?" if this typically results in receiving a glass of water. This becomes more complex when a statement such as "I just want to die," acquires a response of listening, care, and statements of affection across settings and across a variety of relationships. If the outcome is just as predictable and reliable as the request for a glass of water, it is similarly a mand.

What, then, does a therapist do with the awareness that the content of one's speech is a result of interactions that do not correspond so neatly to concepts such as accuracy of reporting, honesty, dishonesty, and rarely can be taken at face value? Consider the woman who says to her partner, "There is no more milk." Is this a description of what she is seeing in the refrigerator? Or is she asking her partner to go to the store? Or is she irritated that her partner forgot to pick up the milk from the store as agreed? Similarly, if a client says, "I don't know what to do!" What does she mean? Is she just describing a state of confusion? Or might this be a prompt for the therapist to offer some suggestions?

Noting that our verbal behavior is a result of learning and may serve a function unrelated to the content of speech is not a statement on the reliability or honesty of any given person. Verbal behavior may have functions of which we are not aware. For example, we may make the statement, "There is no more milk" unaware that we are requesting our partner to go to the store.

With verbal behavior (i.e., speaking, thinking, writing), the possibility of hidden functions (i.e., hidden meaning) is especially significant. Our clients sometimes say more with their words than is apparent. The behavioral notion of function provides a useful tool for unpacking this wisdom and systematically inquiring into the complexity of language (Kohlenberg & Tsai, 1991; Tsai et al., 2009). A full behavior analysis would evaluate the context in which the statement was made to address the question, "What function did the statement serve?" Why was it said now and not earlier or later? Where was it said? What happened right after it was said? What happened earlier in the histories of the speaker and listener relevant to this event? Thus, an entire narrative is wrapped around the single statement, "There is no more milk." We might imagine numerous stories in which the same statement occurs. Daily life is full of examples of statements with obvious hidden meanings, such as when a teenager says sarcastically, "Wow, thank you for enlightening me!" or a neighbor, panting as he lifts a dresser up his front steps, comments, "Man, this is really heavy." These hidden meanings, as noted, are relatively obvious and both speaker and listener are aware of the multiple meanings.

A crucial point for the FAP therapist to keep in mind, however, is that hidden meanings of therapeutic interest may not be deliberate or conscious. The client who, when confused, says, "I don't know what to do!" and stares plaintively at her therapist while her mind goes blank and panic crawls up her belly, may not be aware that when she has repeatedly shared confusion with important others in the past, they have jumped into action for her. Thus, she now favors sharing confusion (and feels increasingly anxious until the other acts) over a range of other possible responses. That is, her statement functions as an indirect or non-deliberate request that the other person act for her. This example can be compared directly to the idea that some suicidal threats, while ostensibly intended to inform the listener of intentions to engage in self-harm, may be covert or hidden cries for help or attention. The function is obtained from the history, in that this was the only way that this person had received such help (reinforcement) from family and caregivers in the past, and they may or may not have conscious awareness of the function or insight into the history that supplied it (i.e., failure of the context to discriminate the function of an individual's behavior).

There is nothing inherently wrong with covert forms of speech, and across cultures, languages differ regarding the relative importance of the content of speech versus contextual cues. This requires the therapist to work with sensitivity toward the culture and context that the client moves through, though the therapist does not need to be a cultural expert to develop hypotheses based upon whether or not the client describes the use of speech that is effective and results in others responding in an expected manner. It is not uncommon, for example, that a client might persist in making statements about their loneliness or desire to connect in a manner that is so frequent and emotive that others find it off-putting and do not respond in a desired manner (CRB1). Ineffective types of speech might be shaped into more effective direct behavior that serves the same function (e.g., asking the therapist for more time or evidence of caring). Similarly, the client who talks about having difficulty cleaning up the garage may be avoiding (a CRB1) directly expressing feelings (likely a CRB2) about being dissatisfied with progress in therapy. In more general terms, exploring hidden meanings resembles the psychoanalytic goal of making the unconscious conscious but, in FAP, it emphasizes using this new awareness to improve interpersonal relating.

In exploring the effectiveness of a client's verbal behavior, and orienting the client toward the function, rather than the content of their ineffective verbal behavior, we encourage our client to orient their awareness toward the impact of their behaviors, rather than their emotional response to ineffective speech.

5

The therapy relationship is a real relationship

We acknowledge that many features of the therapy situation are artificial, for example, meeting once a week at a specific time for 45 minutes, fee for service, boundaries such as not having contact outside the therapy room with clients, and prohibitions against physical intimacy. On the other hand, if we use our behavioral lens to examine what actually is "real" about the therapy relationship, we turn to functional analysis to understand the meaning of the term "real." What is "real" in the therapy relationship is defined as that which evokes the same responses that are evoked in daily life relationships—that is, the situations are functionally the same. For example, the typical therapy setting is defined by two people who come together to talk about the problems of one of the discussants. By its very nature, the therapy setting is an interpersonal context that requires risk-taking, disclosure, trust, and honesty; therefore, it contains all of the stimuli associated with evaluation, rejection, and social punishment, in addition to the stimuli associated with the emotional closeness of being attended to and cared about. Similarly, therapy relationships have beginnings and endings. Thus, if the client's daily life issues have to do with intimacy, risk-taking, disclosure, trust, rejection, beginnings, and endings, and these issues are evoked in the therapist-client relationship, functional analysis would indicate that the therapy relationship is "real" in these domains. By the same token, if the therapy relationship is functionally the same in this way, generalization would be expected to occur (Tsai et al., 2019).

Clients sometimes will say they cannot emotionally connect, be open, vulnerable, or be therapeutically intimate with the therapist due to artificial boundaries such as the common limits regarding time and frequency of sessions. Although this might be a valid objection, it is important for the FAP therapist to maintain a functional perspective. For example, if the client's daily life problem has to do with forming intimate relationships, the functional similarity (reality) between therapy and outside relationships is that all relationships (both inside and outside of therapy) have limitations and boundaries. The client's CRBs might include not taking the risks that are necessary to connect and deal with the limitations and disappointments inherent in all relationships.

We have focused here on how to apply functional analysis to account for and assess those areas in which the therapy relationship is real (i.e., the "same" as daily life). We should also point out that FAP includes interventions and suggestions on how to enhance the functional equivalence or the reality of the therapist-client relationship. FAP therapists are encouraged (in the therapy context with their clients' target behaviors in mind) to be their real selves, to self-disclose, to be genuine, to express positive feelings, and to be courageous and therapeutically loving in both evoking and naturally reinforcing client behavior. Similarly, FAP therapists generally eschew using standardized "one size fits all" interventions and limit the use of role-playing, behavioral rehearsal, or social skills training because these methods pose the risk of being artificial and might decrease functional equivalence (realness). Furthermore, once CRB2s take place in the therapy relationship, FAP offers guidance in helping to transfer gains from the therapist-client relationship to the client's daily life.

6

The central role of natural reinforcement

Consider the following questions that a client might ask: "Why am I the way that I am?", "Why do I seem to get into such destructive relationships?", "Why am I so self-critical?", "Why do I have such low self-esteem?", "Why am I preoccupied with thoughts and plans to kill myself?" There is, of course, an almost endless list of questions of this type.

Now let us say that you as a therapist are going to answer, but you are limited to a brief response, and further, your answer will be informed by a behavioral perspective. The answer then is, "because of the contingencies of reinforcement you have experienced." Needless to say, if you actually did give this answer, your client would most likely be utterly confused and perhaps consider getting another therapist. Further, without a more in-depth understanding of what is meant by "reinforcement," many therapists would consider the answer to be theoretically deficient. Nevertheless, this is the answer that underlies a core view of FAP, and once fully understood, it will be very useful in guiding your therapeutic work.

In this point, we will spell out the essence of what is meant by reinforcement; in later points, we will discuss how this idea is put to practical use to intensify your therapeutic work and improve outcomes, regardless of the type of therapy you do (see Chapter 22). By definition, *contingencies of reinforcement* are consequences—how the world, including both the physical and interpersonal world, responds to behavior—and at any given moment, the world is either strengthening (reinforcing) or not strengthening (punishing or extinguishing) a person's behavior by supplying consequences.

Contingencies of reinforcement are important because they are primary causes of our actions, which include everything that we do such as thinking, believing, noticing, perceiving, walking, eating, expressing feelings, and hiding feelings. Nevertheless, the importance of contingencies of reinforcement is frequently overlooked in therapist-client interactions occurring throughout the therapy session.

Contingency means that when you act in a certain way, your action produces an effect or consequence. Often these effects occur in the physical world; for example, turning the ignition on in your car has the effect of starting the engine. Because this book is about helping clients, however, and almost all client problems involve interpersonal relating, the effects or consequences we focus on are the ways that others react to your interpersonal or social behavior. When you act in a certain way, and the effect that your action has on others makes it more or less likely that you will act in the same way in the future, the effect is referred to as a contingency of reinforcement. There are a few nuances, however, to the preceding statement. When the consequence makes it more likely that you will act in the same way again, it is called *positive reinforcement*. When the consequence makes it less likely that you will act in the same way again, it is called *punishment*. When there is no longer a consequence for an action that was positively reinforced in the past, you are less likely to keep acting that way. Your behavior will stop, and this effect is referred to as *extinction*.

Reinforcement is among one of the most studied and empirically evaluated concepts in psychology (Williams, 1983). Keep in mind, however, that "reinforcement" is just a word. Like any other word, it is understood from the context within which it is used. As used in FAP, reinforcement can be of great assistance to achieving the goals of psychotherapy regardless of the theoretical approach. Reinforcement has two important qualities that when understood can help further its application as a broad principle: reinforcement is ubiquitous, and it typically occurs without awareness.

It is important to highlight that contingencies of reinforcement can be natural or arbitrary. *Natural reinforcement* implies consequences that already occur in the environment and strengthen a large and variable set of responses, while *arbitrary reinforcement* involves consequences set by a specific context (e.g., parents, groups, partners) that mainly benefit from the individual's behaviors but might not serve the individual's interaction with other sources of reinforcement (Ferster, 1967b). The distinction between natural and arbitrary reinforcement is crucial in FAP implementation. FAP therapists seek to promote interpersonal repertoires in-session that can be transferred outside of the session. To increase the chances of generalization (see Chapter 17), therapists must provide natural reinforcement to clients' CRB2s. If therapists provide arbitrary reinforcement, they might hinder the client's chances of encountering reinforcement for their progress in other relationships.

One way to understand reinforcement in our moment-to-moment daily experiences is through the lens of a behaviorist who views the stream of our actions and consequences from a reinforcement standpoint. Our current behavior is a function of the history of reinforcements that have shaped it in the past, just as the strength, width, and shape of a stream at any one point are a function of the topography of the mountain from which it flowed. It is also crucial to fully understand the social dynamic and cultural practices that forge clients' environments. As we are behaving, reinforcement is constantly occurring, shaping our stream, and making certain actions more likely and others less likely. Our future behavior, when it occurs, is a product of this history and socio-cultural contingencies.

Typically, reinforcement has little to do with whether we are aware of having positive feelings after a particular action. A child learning to walk is not aware that each successful landing of a step reinforces the taking of it; a student learning to read may not be aware that each day the behavior is becoming more successful and thereby stronger; a professor who provides the same lecture year after year may or may not be aware of how student reactions have shaped his style and delivery into what it is; a couple in a long, satisfying marriage may not be aware of how exquisitely sensitive and responsive to each other they have become. A reinforcement perspective has been used to account for almost every aspect of human activity, including language, literature, and creativity (Skinner, 1957); spirituality (Hayes, 1984); personality (Bolling et al., 2006); and intimacy and attachment (Kohlenberg et al., 2009).

Taking awareness away from the process of reinforcement means that the primary way to determine if reinforcement has occurred is to observe future occurrences of the behavior. One may also refer to a non-behavioral system: the neurobiological changes that take place when reinforcement has occurred. Our bodies, however, do not have the appropriate sensory systems in the brain for detecting these subtle neurobiological changes when they occur. Synapses and pathways simply are strengthened. Certainly, sometimes in the moment, we may feel pleased and if asked, we might say we are likely to act this way again in the future. But this feeling is not reinforcement nor is it necessary to have this feeling in order to be reinforced.

Thus, reinforcement can be seen as an ongoing and ubiquitous process that does not exclude any aspect of human experience. Our clients' life problems can be viewed as the result of a history of contingencies of reinforcement, and psychotherapy can be seen as an opportunity to provide contingencies of reinforcement to enhance our clients' productive and fulfilling lives.

7

Clinically relevant behaviors (CRBs)

At every moment during the therapy session, your clients are behaving. Some of these behaviors are obvious, such as listening to you, making eye contact, talking, being silent, thinking about what they are going to say next, and expressing anger. Some behaviors are less obvious, such as feeling (e.g., emotions like fear, sadness, love, worthlessness, rejection), perceiving (e.g., that you are concerned), interpreting, avoiding being in the moment, and emotionally withdrawing. If you can adopt the view that nearly everything a client does in session is behavior, then any particular moment in therapy opens up the possibility for you to be reinforcing. Out of the universe of possible behaviors to reinforce, we refer to a select subsample of behavior as clinically relevant behaviors (CRBs). They are called "clinically relevant" because they meet the same function as behaviors that occur in clients' daily lives that have brought them into therapy.

In some cases, CRBs are obvious. For example, a client who gets anxious and cannot think clearly when interacting with an authority figure has the very same problem with the therapist. In other cases, however, CRBs are identified functionally, and this is not at all obvious. For example, consider that a client's daily life relationship problems are the result of a tendency to inappropriately view love and caring expressed by a close partner as not being genuine (e.g., a "trust" issue). This client similarly thinks the therapist is expressing kindness and caring because s/he is "paid" to. Because of the difference between a close partner and a therapist, one might say these are not the same behaviors. But as described in Chapter 3, behavior is defined functionally, by context and meaning. In this case the behavior of interest is "trusting" others to be sincere and honest. From a functional standpoint, the trust behavior that occurs in the client's close relationship also occurs in the relationship with the therapist and thus is a CRB.

DOI: 10.4324/9781032694832-8

Some might recognize the resemblance between this notion of CRB and the psychoanalytic notion of *transference* where the patient transfers their neurosis to the therapist. To be sure, FAP posits that the client's daily life problems may occur in the context of the relationship with the therapist but, unlike psychoanalysis, CRBs are viewed as the result of normal, nonpathological stimulus generalization from daily life to the therapy relationship. In other words, in FAP, the client-therapist relationship is a real relationship.

There are three types of CRB, and understanding the distinction among these is central to doing FAP. CRB1s are client problems that occur in session and meet similar functions as problems outside of session. The trusting and speech anxiety examples given above are examples of CRB1s. To be clear, a client talking about trust or difficulties with authorities is not CRB. CRB1s actually occur in the here and now—"trusting problems" or "speaking anxiety problems" in relation to the therapist. CRB1s are by definition related to the client's presenting problems and often involve emotional avoidance, such as conceling informationand having difficulty expressing honest feelings or personal wants to the therapist. The daily life manifestations of these problems involve shutting down, making indirect comments to get what s/he wants, and disguising his/her feelings in relationships with intimate partners, parents, coworkers, and friends. An example would be a depressed individual who feels controlled by his wife and is passive in his relationship with her, and who shows up session after session with nothing to contribute to the therapy agenda, passively accepting whatever the therapist suggests.

CRB2s are client improvements (skillful behaviors) that occur in session. Early in FAP, CRB2s do not occur or are quite weak (this would be expected since CRB1s are of higher strength). A common theme for most therapists is to encourage clients to reveal innermost feelings that are typically avoided, such as fear, rejection, and love for the therapist. Concealing, cutting oneself off from, or withholding these feelings from the therapist might be a commonly occurring CRB1. In those cases when emotional avoidance is a CRB1, expressing and having feelings about the therapy or therapist would be a CRB2. Similarly, in those cases where the clients' daily life problem is not asking others for what they want, the CRB1 would similarly not be making requests of the therapist. Examples of parallel CRB2s might include asking for a reduced fee, requesting a change in the appointment time, or asking the therapist for a genuine impression about the client.

Note that the definition of CRB2 pivots on the word "improvement." In order to know whether a CRB2 has occurred, it is first important to know what the baseline CRB1 looks like. For example, consider the client who frequently and abruptly quits therapy without offering any explanation as to what precipitated this—a definite CRB1. After a number of CRB1 quits, this client, for the first time, told the therapist that she was quitting therapy because there was too long a period between therapy sessions. The therapist astutely recognized this latter quit as a CRB2 because an explanation was given and reinforced the client by suggesting ways they could have shorter but more frequent visits.

CRB3s are client interpretations of behavior, which are frequent in session. Clients will often ask therapists for interpretations of their own behavior (e.g., "Why do I get so anxious when I try to assert myself?"). From a FAP standpoint, the preferred explanation is a more functional one that refers to histories of reinforcement and punishment. For example, if a client says, "I get anxious because I don't believe I am a worthy person," the therapist might encourage a more functional interpretation such as, "While growing up, whenever I attempted to assert myself or ask for what I wanted I was criticized, and thus punished, and, incidentally, I also felt worthless." The more functional interpretation is preferred because it points to a therapeutic solution, for example, "take a chance and ask for what you would like and see if you get punished or not." Functional interpretations also serve clients' generalization of CRBs outside therapy and discrimination of reinforcing vs. punishing contexts (see Chapter 24).

A failure to make the CRB1 versus CRB2 distinction can lead to counter-therapeutic interventions. Consider a therapist who was using CBT and relaxation to help a client overcome a fear of being assertive with her husband. After several weeks of this work, the therapist suggested they do a role-play in which the therapist would act out the role of the husband by demanding that the client iron his shirts and that she was then to practice role-playing assertiveness. The client politely refused to do the role-playing because it seemed too artificial to her. The therapist failed to recognize that this was a significant CRB2 of being assertive with the therapist (the desired goal for her and her husband) and told her she apparently did not fully understand the prior CBT and relaxation training, and so they would repeat this until she was more amenable to doing a role-play. No doubt the therapist had good intentions, but inadvertently missed a significant therapeutic opportunity, and even worse, punished a CRB2. The therapist's response was thus counter-therapeutic.

At the beginning of this chapter, we noted that the distinction between the types of CRBs is central to doing FAP. It is considered counter-therapeutic to inadvertently punish CRB2s and reinforce CRB1s. Effective FAP involves shaping, nurturing, and reinforcing CRB2s (Tsai et al., 2016).

8

Interpersonal repertories: The core of FAP intervention

We as humans are a social species. We have moved from surviving to thriving by building up communities that rely on social agreements about what is the most beneficial way of interacting with one another. Our social group became a vital source for our subsistence and well-being; and therefore, our ability to establish and maintain valuable social relationships is a fundamental repertoire. However, the changes we have undergone through our lifestyle and social dynamics such as the cult of individualism, the constant demands for productivity, and the fast pace of life have shortened the opportunities to develop interpersonal skills needed to thrive in groups and socially connect. Humans are living in a paradox. In an era of hyperconnectivity, we have never felt more alone. Our basic needs (e.g., social connection) and current context (e.g., social environment) pull in different directions, shaping interpersonal repertoires that seem contradictory in some aspects (i.e., sharing intimate information with strangers on social networks while concealing it from those closest ones) and underdeveloped in others (i.e., having skills to start an interaction, but not to maintain a friendship).

FAP is an intervention focused on shaping and modeling interpersonal repertoires that aid individuals in thriving in the social world. The social nature of therapeutic relationships in this therapy facilitates the transformation of social processes central to human functioning such as affiliation and attachment, socio-emotional communication, and perspective-taking (Cuthbert & Insel, 2013). In FAP sessions, therapists are focused on evoking and reinforcing clients' interpersonal repertoires in order to favor interpersonal competencies, defined as "the ability of a person to interact effectively with other people" (Spitzberg & Cupach, 1989, p. 1).

DOI: 10.4324/9781032694832-9

Callaghan (2006a) developed the Functional Idiographic Assessment Template (FIAT), a behaviorally oriented framework designed to guide therapists when seeking to enhance interpersonal competencies. He suggested that the therapeutic relationship is the setting in which therapists can actively shape and model effective interpersonal repertoires, particularly (a) Assertion of needs, (b) Bidirectional communication, (c) Conflicts management, (d) Disclosure and interpersonal closeness, and (e) Emotional experience and expression.

The FIAT delineates each class of interpersonal functioning with a thorough description of behavioral repertoires and the controlling factors targeted to bolster people's interpersonal competencies (see Chapter 20 for more details on how to notice them in session). Follette et al. (2000) introduced a functional framework to categorize clinical issues from a behavior-analytic viewpoint. They claimed that behavioral problems were related to difficulties in antecedent control (i.e., stimulus control), the responses, or the consequential control (i.e., functional classes). While FIAT focuses on the antecedents and responses involved in interpersonal problems (Callaghan, 2006a), issues of consequential control are equally pivotal within the interpersonal realm. Often, difficulties arise from the consequences (reinforcers) encountered in social interactions, which may be inadequate, of low quality, or in conflict with concurrent consequences (Follette et al., 2000). Table 8.1 offers a comprehensive overview of the interpersonal competencies identified by FIAT, categorized by functional domains of interest. This table outlines possible issues within each domain, serving as a guideline for therapists to navigate a range of interpersonal difficulties faced by clients. Although extensive, this list is not exhaustive; therapists might recognize additional competencies and problems beyond those mentioned. The intent of providing this list is to facilitate, not constrain, your analytical process. As such, therapists should feel confident to provide a stand-alone process-based FAP intervention for those in need of thriving in the social world.

Table 8.1 FIAT interpersonal competencies, functional domains, and processes targeted

Competency (Skillful classes of behavior)	Problems in antecedents control	Problems in behavioral repertoires	Problems in consequential control	Processes
Class A: Assertion of needs	• Difficulty in identifying cues and behaviors that facilitate the communication of needs and boundaries. • Inappropriate discriminative control of communication of needs/opinions/desires/boundaries.	• Excessive/Interfering communication of needs/opinions/desires/boundaries. • Low rate of communication of needs/opinions/desires/boundaries.	• Avoidance of needs/opinions/desires/boundaries. • Obtaining inappropriate or poor positive reinforcement for communicating needs/opinions/desires/boundaries • Competing consequences that interfere with communicating needs/opinions/desires/boundaries.	• Socio-emotional communication.
Class B: Bidirectional communication	• Difficulty noticing the other's perspective. • Difficulty noticing their own perspective. • Difficulty noticing the impact of their own behavior on others or others' behaviors on themselves. • Inappropriate discriminative control to communicate their own perspective or others perspective.	• Excessive/Interfering communication of their own perspective (self-references) or others' perspective. • Low rate of communication of their own perspective or others' perspective. • Low rate of reciprocity.	• Tendency to avoid sharing their own perspective. • Obtaining inappropriate or poor positive reinforcement for communicating their own perspective or others' perspective. • Competing consequences that interfere with communicating their own perspective.	• Perspective-taking.

(Continued)

Table 8.1 (*Continued*)

Competency (Skillful classes of behavior)	Problems in antecedents control	Problems in behavioral repertoires	Problems in consequential control	Processes
Class C: Conflicts management	• Difficulty noticing factors that trigger conflicts. • Inappropriate discriminative control of conflicts. • Difficulty recognizing the effects of their disagreement on others.	• Excessive/Interfering communication of disagreements. • Low rate of communication disagreements. • Limited use of negotiation strategies.	• Avoidance of conflicts or disagreements. • Obtaining inappropriate or poor positive reinforcement for revealing disagreements. • Competing consequences that interfere with communicating disagreements.	• Socio-emotional communication. • Perspective-taking.
Class D: Disclosure and interpersonal closeness	• Difficulty noticing contextual cues that foster vulnerability/intimacy/social connection. • Inappropriate discriminative control of vulnerability/intimacy/social connection. • Difficulty noticing the impact of their vulnerability on others. • Difficulty noticing sources of reinforcement for intimacy.	• Excessive/Interfering communication of vulnerability. • Low rate of communication of vulnerability. • Low rate of engagement in intimate interactions.	• Avoidance of close relationships/vulnerability/intimacy. • Obtaining inappropriate or poor positive reinforcement for vulnerability/intimacy. • Competing consequences that interfere with vulnerability/intimacy/social connection.	• Affiliation and attachment. • Perspective-taking.
Class E: Emotional experience and expression	• Difficulty noticing private contextual cues that signal affect or emotions. • Difficulty noticing public contextual cues for emotional communication. • Difficulty discriminating contexts that favor emotional communication.	• Excessive/Interfering communication of emotions • Excessive/Interfering emotional experience. • Low rate of emotional communication.	• Avoidance of emotional experience/communication • Obtaining inappropriate or poor positive reinforcement for communicating emotions. • Competing consequences that interfere with emotional communication/experience.	• Socio-emotional communication

9

Emotions and feelings

Clients' emotions and feelings play a critical role in FAP. Our approach to this topic, however, is different from most other therapies. The difference in perspective is in (a) our explanation of what feelings are, (b) our assertion that feelings and emotions do not cause problematic behavior, but avoidance of them often does, and (c) our account of why it is important for our clients to be emotional during the therapy session (Kuei et al., 2018)

In FAP, the term "feeling" is really two words, each with a distinct meaning. One meaning of feeling is as a verb, and the other is as a noun. When used as a verb, feeling is an activity, a type of sensory action, such as seeing or hearing. (Yes, to the behaviorist, "seeing" is a behavior; it is something we do and is shaped by contingencies of reinforcement.) When it is a noun, a feeling (also referred to as an emotion) is the object that is felt, as in "I feel (verb) a feeling (noun)."

What is the object being felt, however, when we feel depressed, anxious, happy, and hopeless? Our behavioral view asserts that what we feel is our body. The "interoceptive" and "proprioceptive" nervous systems are involved in the body feeling process. These two nervous systems are stimulated by the parts of the body involved in fear, anger, depression, anxiety, joy, and the like.

How does the body get in that particular state which is then felt? It is the result of our unique learning history (operant and respondent conditioning and associated verbal processes). The important point here is that we view the external environment as the ultimate cause of the bodily states associated with feelings such as fear, anger, hurt, and love. Just because the bodily state is present, however, does not mean one is aware of or can describe feelings.

We are not born knowing what our emotions are any more than we are born knowing (or even noticing) what a ball is. These must be taught by adults, mainly our parents and caretakers. In the case of feelings, the object being felt (the body) is private, and the parent or adult who is trying to teach a child to be aware of and identify feelings is at a disadvantage. In contrast to teaching the child to sense (see) a ball, the adult can point to the ball, pronounce its name, and reinforce a response such as "ball." Thus, it is not surprising there is confusion about what we feel. Nor is it surprising for a client to look puzzled and say, "I don't know" when asked, "What are you feeling right now?" In addition to being confused about labeling (or even being aware) of feelings, the expression or showing of feelings is often punished in our culture because we place substantial prohibitions on displays of emotion (Nichols & Efran, 1985). The net result is that many client problems involve difficulties due to: (a) identifying and/or describing feelings, (b) avoiding situations that evoke negative (or positive) feelings, and (c) not being aware (cut off) from feelings or "numbing."

In the service of being aware of and evoking CRBs (Rules 1 and 2, see Chapter 20), you can offer your clients a behavioral rationale for getting in touch with feelings and for being emotional during the therapy session. FAP therapists underscore that the importance of being emotional in session is *not* based on the benefits of cathartic release (e.g., "It's good to get it out, to release those bottled-up feelings," or "If you hold them back they will come out in some other way"). Instead, the rationale is that avoiding feelings has a cost. Avoiding feelings is accomplished through reduced awareness of one's own internal (bodily) states, one's external (interpersonal) environment, and deliberate avoidance of feeling-evocative situations (e.g., keeping a distance from a potentially intimate relationship). Thus, the absence of emotion interferes with therapy, and correspondingly, with other areas of daily life. Emotional expression is crucial because it serves as a marker that clients are in touch with themselves and the world and provides them the opportunity to learn how to act in new ways that improve their lives. For example, we might say to a client who is avoiding grieving over a relationship that has ended:

> It's important to let yourself grieve, because if you avoid thinking, feeling, and talking about your ex, then you may end up avoiding those activities that you once did together, or meeting new people

who might evoke the same feelings you had for your ex. Even worse, you might end up cutting off awareness of private feelings of attraction and connection. By avoiding all these things, not only is the richness of your life interfered with, but you also lose the opportunity to figure out what went wrong and to learn new ways of dealing with someone close to you when similar problems come up.

Another intervention that can help reduce emotional avoidance is to re-present, in the session, the situation that evokes the avoidance (CRB1). For example, when clients have difficulty accepting care from others (the avoidance of expressions of caring feelings by others) and need help in getting in touch with and expressing their feelings, especially feelings of closeness, we encourage an active expression of feelings by therapists concerning their care for and connection to the client.

In accordance with Rule 3 (see Chapter 22), a therapist's response to displays of emotion ideally should be naturally reinforcing to encourage reductions in emotional avoidance and to set the scene for therapeutic progress. A therapist who has difficulty with his/her own or with others' affective expression is unlikely to offer such encouragement and may inadvertently punish a client's contact with or expression of affect. Someone with this type of deficient repertoire clearly would be less able to work well with clients who require increased contact with stimuli evoking emotional responses. Therefore, therapists should strive to increase their awareness and be willing to work on dealing with their own issues, such as exploring their own avoidance repertoires, so that they can more effectively help their clients address feelings.

Development and support of the self

Like emotions and feelings, the *self* figures prominently in many clients' presenting problems: "I have no self-esteem," "I don't know who I am," "I want to find my true self," or "My family says I have not been myself lately." The *self*, in fact, has been a salient topic in the history of psychotherapy, and many theories of the *self* have been advanced (Deikman, 1973; Erikson, 1968; Kohut, 1971; Masterson, 1985).

Given a renewed interest in the self within ACT, drawing upon relational frame theory, or the inner workings of the self in approaches such as compassion-focused therapy (CFT), this should not be as surprising as it may once have been. While one can be aware of the experience of a sense of self, much like one might experience the taste of salt, it may not be obvious how such experiences have been learned.

What is the *self*? For many individuals, the self is that which has been present across all other experiences. What one thinks, sees, feels, wants, and so forth, will vary across time, but the experience of one's self is of something stable, a constant perspective from which thinking, seeing, feeling, and wanting occur. One does not experience a sense of difference in the self that sees their reflection in a mirror, day after day, year after year. Learning to orient toward or label that experience, however, is a learned behavior, so like any other, the quality of instruction may vary, and problems can occur.

Consider a child learning to name a ball. When the child says "ball" in the presence of an actual ball, the parent or caregiver will demonstrate excitement or offer praise, providing reinforcement for the correct label. When the child says "ball" when the object referred to is not a ball, the parent will correct or ignore the child. In this way, over repeated instances of such training and through other behavioral processes beyond the scope of this example (Hayes et al., 2001), the child learns to correctly identify balls. The training is relatively simple because it is easy for parents to gauge whether the child is correct in saying "ball" by ascertaining that a ball is present.

DOI: 10.4324/9781032694832-11

Now consider a child learning to name "hunger." As with ball, we want the child to say "hunger" (or a functional equivalent, like "I want food," "food," "eat," or "hungry") in the presence of the experience of hunger and not in the presence of other experiences. The parental task here is undoubtedly more difficult than in the case of the ball. Hunger is much harder to identify because it is a private experience, not a public object to which the parent has easy visual or tactile access. The parent may notice the length of time since the child's last meal, how much the child has been eating lately, or the child's irritable mood and suggest, "You must be hungry." Sensitive parents, of course, successfully meet this challenge most of the time, but even the most attuned parents will not be as accurate with "hunger" as they will be with "ball." Other parents may disregard a child's attempt to name private experiences such as hunger or sadness, punish those attempts when inconvenient, or weaken accurate labeling through only positively responding when the child's description of an inner state matches their own experiences. Thus, one's experience of self may be accurate and confident, or inaccurate, confused, and dependent on others. Essentially, one may say with accuracy and confidence, "I know who I am," or one may say, "I don't know who I am." According to this theory, severe problems with the self, as in those experienced by clients diagnosed with borderline personality disorder or disorders of the self (e.g., dissociative identity disorder), are a function of severely disordered, neglectful, traumatic, and invalidating instruction with respect to private experiences (Kohlenberg & Tsai, 1991).

Relational frame theory, a model of verbal learning, elaborates on this process of learning to label private events (e.g., Montoya-Rodríguez et al., 2017). In this model, one does not only internalize the distinction between "I" and "you," but also learns the distinction between "here" and "there" as a quality of the embodied experience of moving through space, and "now" and "then" resulting from the awareness of the passage of time. This model incorporates perspective-taking into a fully developed self. This creates more opportunities for the creative therapist to strengthen a client's weak sense of self, perhaps through encouraging what one's 7-year-old self might say to their adult self. It also describes additional ways that one's experience of the self might be invalidated, such as when a family member continues to respond to one according to their tastes or habits when they were a child, not acknowledging the passage of time. Common FAP interactions in therapy rely upon movement across these dimensions, such as shifting along the I-you axis ("What do you imagine I feel toward you in this moment?"), the here-there relationship ("What would you say if she were in front of you right now?"), or the now-then axis ("What will the you of five years from now think of this moment in your life?"). The self is, in this way, not just a "thing" as much as a form of engagement with the world, and the variety of ways that we engage in *selfing* are deeply connected to how we experience others and develop empathy.

Thus, the FAP therapist sees no theoretical obstacles to working on problems of the self, and in fact employs a theoretical stance that may clarify the work to be done. Self-experiences may be conceptualized as varying on a continuum from complete private control over the experience (resulting in accurate and confident self-expressions) to complete public control (resulting in absent, inaccurate, confused, or dependent self-expressions). The therapeutic task is to shape private control over the experience, and functionally the therapeutic hour affords many opportunities to do so. Agenda setting, provision of homework, simple questions, even therapeutic misunderstandings, all may be seen as opportunities to evoke and reinforce client self-expression. In FAP, problems with the experience of self become CRB1s, and a full set of FAP techniques can be used to address and transform these issues (Kohlenberg et al., 2009).

11

Cognitions and beliefs

As a behavioral therapy approach, how does FAP address cognitions and beliefs? Many individuals without a behavioral background may have learned that behaviorists deny the existence of cognition and belief, that anything inside the "black box" of the mind that cannot be observed does not exist.

This characterization of behaviorism has no relation to FAP. FAP takes everything that a client does—acting, thinking, believing, loving, feeling, hoping, and so forth—seriously. Behaviorists do not deny mental experiences; they do eschew treating those experiences as entities to explain other experiences. For example, cognitive theory posits that cognitive structures such as schemas give rise to specific automatic thoughts as well as overt behaviors (Clark et al., 1999). While behaviorists argue that cognitive structures or schemas do not exist, they are very interested in the experience and process of thinking and in thoughts.

A trickier issue is whether thoughts cause behavior, and behaviorists over the years have been somewhat inconsistent on this issue. The first obstacle to viewing thoughts as causes was pragmatic in that traditionally, behaviorists preferred to locate causes in the environment because environmental conditions are presumably manipulable. Early behavioral interventions, however, sometimes included behavioral thought-stopping interventions, and modern cognitive therapists might reasonably argue that the techniques of cognitive therapy are quite effective at changing thoughts. Thus, the argument that thoughts are not manipulable is not very convincing in today's psychotherapeutic environment.

The second argument against viewing thoughts as causes was theoretical. Because thinking is seen as a behavior, it is theoretically problematic for the behaviorist to suggest that one behavior (thinking) causes another behavior, as we want to look outside the behavioral system for causes of behavior. Both traditional behavioral accounts, however, of language and cognition (Skinner, 1957) and more recent accounts (Hayes et al., 2001) make it clear that thoughts, as private events, can have stimulus properties such as eliciting and evocative functions. In other words, what one thinks can influence how one feels and what one does. From a FAP perspective, any behaviorist who denies that thinking can have an impact on behavior is being unnecessarily dogmatic. Thus, today's behaviorism includes rich and sophisticated accounts of language and cognition and how they influence overt behavior (Hayes & Brownstein, 1986).

Equally dogmatic as the behaviorist who denies the role of cognition, from a FAP perspective, is a cognitivist who demands that all clinically relevant overt behavior must have cognitive causes. In FAP, sometimes thinking has an impact on behavior, and sometimes it does not (Kohlenberg et al., 2010). FAP, while allowing for the possibility that thinking may influence behavior, retains a behavioral worldview that explores the individual's historical and current context as the determinants of the relation between thinking and behavior. This suggests that whether thinking impacts behavior may vary from time to time depending on other contextual factors.

For example, consider a client with recurrent panic attacks. The client reports that the panic attack was triggered by getting on the bus, and when asked if s/he had any panic-related thoughts while getting on the bus, s/he reports "Yes, I remember thinking that I was trapped and that I could not easily get off the bus if I had to, and then very soon after that I started feeling panic." In this case, it is possible that the client's thinking was influential with respect to triggering the panic. Thus, the traditional cognitive A-B-C model, in which A represents an antecedent event (getting on the bus), B represents an intervening belief or cognition ("I feel trapped"), and C represents the emotional consequence (panic), would apply, and a FAP therapist might usefully employ this model as part of treatment.

Cognitive and FAP therapists would respond differently, however, if in response to the question about panic-related thoughts while getting on the bus, the client reported, "I was not aware of any. The panic just came on as soon as I sat down on the bus. Actually, I was thinking about my work." A cognitive therapist dogmatically adhering to the A-B-C model would possibly continue to explore automatic thoughts that occurred quickly in that situation and precipitated the panic, explaining that the thoughts may happen so fast that the client does not notice them, but upon reflection, they logically must be there. The FAP therapist would probably not do this, because our model allows for the possibility that the panic can be triggered directly by getting on the bus with no intervening thoughts.

Furthermore, there are other possibilities. For example, getting on the bus could cause both panic-related thoughts and panic symptoms simultaneously. In other words, the panic thoughts occurred, but they did not participate in causing the panic. Alternately, getting on the bus could directly cause the panic symptoms, then the symptoms caused the thoughts. This would be an A-C-B model (Kanter et al., 2004). The bottom line is that the behavioral worldview upon which FAP is based is very flexible and sees the traditional A-B-C model as just one of many possible options for the relation between thinking and feeling.

Therapeutically, this opens up many interventions to the FAP therapist. When the A-B-C model applies, the techniques of Cognitive Therapy (e.g., Beck et al., 1979) may be used by FAP therapists to challenge thoughts. In fact, considerable theoretical and empirical work has been devoted to adding FAP techniques to those of Cognitive Therapy, resulting in a treatment called FAP-Enhanced Cognitive Therapy, or FECT (R. J. Kohlenberg et al., 2002). In FECT, therapists assess, on a situation-by-situation basis, whether the A-B-C model applies. When it does, they employ cognitive techniques, although while doing so, as FAP therapists, they are alert to opportunities to shift into FAP processes when CRBs occur.

Even in cases where the A-B-C model applies, however, additional considerations may be useful before the FAP therapist engages in cognitive restructuring *per se*. First, even in cases when thoughts are causally related to clinically relevant behavior, behavioral research and theory (Hayes et al., 1999) suggest that challenging thoughts as per traditional cognitive therapy may not be the best or most useful approach (Longmore & Worrell, 2007). Instead, the FAP therapist may choose to help the client accept and defuse from the thoughts, rather than working directly at changing their content, as per the techniques of ACT. Several published discussions and case studies of integrating FAP and ACT (FACT) are available (Baruch et al., 2009a; Callaghan et al., 2004; B. S. Kohlenberg & Callaghan, 2010).

Although FECT has been shown to be promising, ACT's acceptance-based approach to thoughts, rather than CT's challenging approach, ultimately may be a better fit with FAP and its worldview for several reasons. First, both ACT and FAP share a common foundation in behaviorism (although ACT has reframed and renamed this philosophy somewhat as *functional contextualism*). Second, in both ACT and FAP, the ultimate goal is behavior change in line with the client's stated goals and values, while CT takes a more medical symptom-reduction approach. Third, both therapies are framed within the PBT umbrella. Finally, the accepting stance of the ACT therapist dovetails nicely with the empathically connected approach of the FAP therapist, while the therapeutic relationship in CT is not as natural a fit with FAP. In fact, ACT techniques often focus the therapist on the here-and-now experience between the client and the therapist, affording easy opportunities to shift into the FAP process while doing ACT.

12

A model for intimacy: Living with awareness, courage, and love (ACL)

Some professionals find the precise and technical language of FAP, based on its radical behavioral roots, to be highly effective, whereas others advocate for more accessible everyday language. Recognizing this diversity in engagement, the rules of FAP were distilled into the more approachable terms of Awareness, Courage, and Love (ACL; Tsai et al., 2013; Tsai et al., 2014). These principles are operationalized as follows: Awareness is cultivated through Noticing (Rule 1), Courage through Evoking (Rule 2), and Love through Reinforcing (Rule 3). The process further emphasizes the significance of recognizing one's impact (Rule 4, further Awareness) and Generalization (Rule 5), which necessitates the harmonious integration of Awareness, Courage, and Love.

As the co-creators of FAP, Robert Kohlenberg and Mavis Tsai grew increasingly alarmed by the global loneliness epidemic and were dismayed to realize that only therapy clients had access to the transformative power of FAP principles. They wanted to share ACL with everyone, not just those who chose or could afford therapy. Thus, the nonprofit organization ACL Global Project was born. Its overarching aim is to democratize access to these powerful principles, extending beyond the therapeutic milieu to address the pervasive public health challenges of loneliness and social isolation. By establishing ACL chapters worldwide, the project aspires to cultivate a global community committed to fostering meaningful relationships and personal authenticity, thereby mitigating loneliness and fostering a culture of openhearted engagement.

The ACL Global Project has evolved into a dynamic international entity, with chapter leaders trained in six continents. It is dedicated to the facilitation of environments conducive to vulnerable self-disclosure and compassionate responsiveness—key elements identified by

DOI: 10.4324/9781032694832-13

research as essential for fulfilling human connections. The project's commitment to evidence-based practice is underscored by ongoing research conducted at the University of Washington. This research encompasses a range of studies, including laboratory evaluations and randomized-controlled trials, aimed at assessing the effectiveness of ACL interventions. Such empirical endeavors serve as the backbone of the project, ensuring that its strategies are informed by scientific evidence (Bowen et al., 2012; Haworth et al., 2015; Hardebeck, 2023; Holman et al., 2012; Kanter et al., 2018; Kohlenberg et al., 2015; Maitland et al., 2024; Pedersen et al., 2024; Tsai et al., 2020).

The ACL Global Project transcends the conventional boundaries of a community; it is a movement propelled by individuals seeking depth, authenticity, and transformative growth. The project emphasizes the importance of genuine, heartfelt interactions as the foundation for personal and collective development. Distinguished by its commitment to research-based initiatives, the project offers a plethora of opportunities for engagement, including collaborative growth platforms, global networking, content creation, and a comprehensive resource library. With a focus on multilingual inclusivity, the community embraces a diverse membership, fostering rich cultural exchanges and the development of authentic selves through a variety of experiential and introspective activities.

By joining the ACL Global Project (https://acl-global-project.mn .co/), individuals contribute their unique perspectives, experiences, and aspirations, enriching the collective narrative and advancing the mission to cultivate a world marked by heightened awareness, courage, and love. This collective endeavor not only addresses the immediate challenges of loneliness and isolation but also lays the groundwork for a future in which every individual feels valued, connected, and empowered to effect positive change.

13

Vulnerability in context

When most people, even many therapists, consider vulnerability and intimacy in the therapeutic relationship, behavior therapy is not what most often springs first to mind. Some of this reputation is deserved, as for decades there were examples of behavior and CBT therapists who approached relationships as external coaches. A difficult relationship might be explored with a thought record, or acronyms introduced that describe principles of effective interactions. Such approaches neglected an important tool that was already available in the room, however: the therapist. As there are already two people present, the possibility to directly shape and reinforce meaningful social behavior is accessible without appeal to reported external events.

Cordova and Scott (2001) elaborated a functional analysis of intimacy and suggested that there are a small number of key contributors that set the stage for the experience of closeness. Specifically, the two dimensions of how infrequently an aspect of one's self or information is revealed, as well as the potential likelihood of rejection, set the stage. Intimacy is not a result of the behavior of only a single actor, however. When an infrequently disclosed part of the self that may lead to rejection occurs, such as when a young non-binary person first comes out to a friend, this information must first be met with warmth by the other. This reinforces the vulnerability that has occurred and becomes a prompting event for the partner in a dyad to then disclose something of similar infrequency and risk. Over time, closeness and intimacy deepen as a result of these exchanges, and of repeatedly behaving in a vulnerable manner that is accepted, reinforced, and mirrored.

This may raise more questions than it answers, initially. While FAP offers a microcosm to experience and try new behaviors within a sacred and intimate space, the degree of reciprocity one might expect in a relationship in daily life would be inappropriate to fully mirror in a therapeutic space. There might also be very sensitive topics that are meaningful and appropriate to share within one's relationships, though are not necessary for the therapist to know (e.g., specific sexual desires or fantasies that might be shared with a romantic partner). A good adage to consider is that the most basic type of authentic and vulnerable disclosure would be to genuinely share how one feels in response to a disclosure made by the client. The addition of specific content from the therapist's life merits deeper consideration.

Therapist self-disclosure

Therapist self-disclosure involves the sharing of information with a client that the client would not normally know or discover. It involves some risk and vulnerability on the part of the therapist and is a key element of FAP as it offers an authentic, natural, and often highly effective means of reinforcing or evoking CRBs and modeling effective behavior.

The notion of strategic use of therapist self-disclosure (Tsai et al., 2010) stands in contrast to early psychotherapy traditions in which therapist anonymity was favored and therapist self-disclosure was considered a breach of the therapeutic frame (Edwards & Murdock, 1994). Since that time, however, theory and a growing body of research have advocated the judicious and strategic use of therapist self-disclosure in certain contexts (e.g., Barrett & Berman, 2001; Knox & Hill, 2003; Watkins, 1990). Interestingly, however, although theory and research support self-disclosure, the literature suggests that it is actually among the most infrequently used therapeutic strategies (Hill et al., 1988). This chapter, therefore, will discuss the rationale behind therapist self-disclosure in FAP, offer some clinical examples of self-disclosure in action, and highlight therapist skills that increase the effectiveness of self-disclosure in session.

When therapists express their personal reactions to CRBs, they provide essential data that clients may never have encountered previously about how their actions impact their relationships and the people around them. When a client's interpersonal behavior improves, the therapist's personal response to this improvement may be a rare and powerful gift given by the therapist to the client. For example, the therapist might say: "The way that you're inviting me to see parts of you and your experience that you rarely share and that you often feel ashamed of is making me feel like I can trust you with vulnerable pieces of myself as well." As clinically indicated based on the case conceptualization, the therapist might go on to disclose specific autobiographical content or other authentic, vulnerable reactions that the therapist is experiencing in response to the client's CRB2. Doing so *may* have the effect of reinforcing the client's disclosure, enhancing the genuine intimacy of the therapeutic relationship, and establishing the therapeutic relationship as more similar to outside relationships, thus facilitating generalization.

Yet, not all clients will find this, or other forms, of self-disclosure reinforcing depending on learning history, the context of the therapy relationship, and the specific interaction with the therapist at any moment. A client with a history of invalidation by meaningful others, who punished self-disclosure and responded warmly only in attempts to attend to their own needs, may result in a client feeling punished by self-disclosure. Hence, it is essential to consistently practice Rule 4, especially when taking risks to disclose increasingly vulnerable content. That said, another potential benefit of self-disclosure is that it gives clients explicit feedback on how the therapist feels and thus provides practice in learning how to read subtle signs indicating how others feel.

Consider a client who originally presented with a depressed mood, panic attacks, social isolation, and a new diagnosis of multiple sclerosis. Initially, the client's attention was understandably consumed by her own suffering, and she relied heavily on the therapist's guidance to function in daily life and to begin taking proactive steps to care for her physical and mental health. In this early phase of treatment, the client's CRB2s included transporting herself independently to sessions and being able to actively collaborate with the therapist in creating homework assignments. These CRB2s were effectively reinforced by therapist self-disclosure in the form of feedback such as: "I can feel more of you here with me when you show up in this active and whole-hearted way as we work together to define what homework is going to be most helpful for you over the course of the week. It inspires me to bring out some more of myself too, including some of my zanier ideas, because I can trust that you'll tell me when they're not the right fit for you." Over time, as the client's sense of self and capacity to care for her own well-being became stronger, her awareness of others had room to begin expanding; therefore, awareness of the therapist became a CRB2 (in service of her outside life goal of deepening interpersonal relationships). The client began noticing more subtle reactions in the therapist and expressing appreciation for elements of the therapist's genuine self that emerged spontaneously in response to her. On one occasion, when the therapist was expressing energetic delight in reaction to a visual metaphor that the client had created, the client said: "I love the way you express enthusiasm! I can see it on your face and hear it in your voice; it makes me feel proud of what I've done and grateful for you." This awareness of the therapist's behavior and its impact on her, as well as the skillful expression of related appreciation, was a clear CRB2 that the therapist reinforced with self-disclosure about the positive impact of the client's gratitude—and so the cycle continued!

Finally, it may be worth noting that, when handled with care, disclosing a negative response to a client CRB1 might be a helpful way to block and evoke a CRB2. For example, in response to a client who describes their experiences in a very dry, clinical manner, a therapist might share,

> I can see how affected you are by the experience you are describing, though I also am not able to feel this emotion with you in a way that would let me into your world. Would you be open to re-telling me about this painful experience without any clinical language or labeling, just what the experience was and what you were feeling?

In this way, a subsequent CRB2 might be evoked that would be reinforced by the therapist's disclosure of genuine empathy and connection.

14

Ethical issues and precautions

FAP seeks to create a deep and profound therapeutic experience; the degree of thoughtfulness, care, and caution that FAP supervisors and therapists bring to their work must be equally deep and profound. Ethical codes developed to guide therapists in general, such as the APA Ethical Guidelines (Ethical Principles of Psychologists and Code of Conduct, 2017 Amendments), are relevant and applicable to FAP. Specific characteristics of FAP ensure some of these guidelines are particularly salient. The following sections delineate areas of potential ethical concern and the ways they relate to FAP. While they emphasize the therapist-client relationship, these issues are equally salient to supervisor-supervisee interactions.

Avoid exploitation

Since the therapy relationship is one of unequal power, it is important to constantly keep in mind the question, "What is best for my client at the moment and in the long run?" Keeping this question at the forefront of treatment minimizes the likelihood of exploiting or harming clients through a host of situations that can be harmful to them: an unhealthy dependence on the therapist, sexual involvement, or interminable treatments where both parties are gratified by a relationship that is more like friendship than therapy. When working with diversity, exploitation is a deeply important matter that is further addressed in Chapter 15.

Understand your client thoroughly

FAP therapists take risks, evoke CRBs, and create intense therapeutic relationships. All these experiences have the potential to be beneficial but also may be stressful and challenging, or even harmful for the client. The therapist therefore must proceed with caution and make careful use of principles of shaping. This requires knowing the client

DOI: 10.4324/9781032694832-15

well, knowing what behaviors exhibited by the therapist will encourage growth and change at a level the client is ready for, and what behaviors will be overwhelming or off-putting in a way that leads to disengagement, undue distress, or even termination of therapy. FAP therapists are encouraged to carefully inform the client of the nature of the treatment (see Chapter 18 on the FAP rationale) and also dose the move into in-session focus in a way that the client can tolerate.

Be controlled by reinforcers that benefit clients

From a FAP perspective, a therapist who is controlled by reinforcers that are not beneficial to the client is a primary source of ethical violations. For example, the therapist may be reinforced by frequent expressions of gratitude and praise from a client for whom such behavior is a CRB1. If the therapist is unaware of this process, they may respond in a manner that reinforces and helps maintain the client's problem. Thus, it is exceedingly important that therapists recognize areas where they may be vulnerable to reinforcers that are not helpful to the client. In such instances, therapist supervision or consultation is always encouraged in FAP.

Increase your self-awareness

FAP encourages therapists to take risks; such risks must be taken in a context of clarity and self-awareness. Effective FAP therapists must have a high level of self-awareness, openness to examining their own motives and reinforcers, and an ability to recognize and respond to their own TIs non-defensively. Although this kind of self-awareness is important for all therapists, we believe it is particularly important in FAP because the therapist is being encouraged to take risks and evoke CRBs. For example, a therapist who is lonely or lacking intimacy in personal relationships may overly rely on therapeutic relationships for a primary source of closeness and be attracted to FAP as a means of increasing or justifying that intimacy. Such a therapist may place demands on the client for greater than appropriate closeness, under the guise of following FAP rules. It is crucial that FAP therapists examine their own responses and TIs in an ongoing way. Again, consultation and supervision are often a crucial part of such exploration.

Have the client's target behavior into your own repertoire

Many clients have difficulty accepting care and help, and have trouble being vulnerable, open, close, or intimate with others. With such clients, the FAP therapist needs to create a context in which there are opportunities to engage with the therapist in new, more connected ways. A therapist who is uncomfortable with closeness and is not addressing that limitation is not likely to engage in behaviors that evoke connection or intimacy sufficiently with their client. The client may not be given the opportunity to work on essential issues around closeness in relationships or be reinforced for CRB2s in this area. Similarly, a therapist who is uncomfortable with intimacy, closeness, or vulnerability may be inclined to interpret a client's request for more connection, personal questions about the therapist, or expressions of reliance on the therapist as CRB1s in a broader class of dependence or neediness in relationships. For some clients, this may be the case, but it is clearly problematic if the therapist's own T1s are leading them to mistakenly assume the client's behavior reflects a CRB1 when it does not.

Alternatively, clients who have difficulty tolerating separation, solitude, or acting independently may need the therapist to help evoke and shape those behaviors. Again, a therapist who has difficulty with distance, autonomy, or separation in relationships may inadvertently reinforce the client's CRB1s. They may not recognize these behaviors as CRB1s or create opportunities for CRB2s to occur.

Do not continue a non-beneficial treatment

FAP-informed treatment does not help all clients. Research also clearly supports the importance of therapist-client match. Having therapy not work well is often emotionally evocative for therapists and can result in problematic behavior such as blaming the client, directly or indirectly distancing from or being rejecting toward the client, becoming overly apologetic, self-critical, or tenaciously continuing therapy without acknowledging the lack of progress. At times, having a client decide not to continue treatment may represent an important CRB2, and FAP therapists must be able to reinforce this behavior.

FAP and multiple relationships

Due to the emotionally intimate and powerful nature of FAP therapy relationships, it is essential to maintain an especially keen awareness of any actual or potential multiple relationships with clients. This genuine, reciprocal emotional intimacy in conjunction with the functionally pragmatic lens of FAP is often a powerful source of healing for clients and yet can also generate confusion regarding what multiple relationships may be acceptable versus harmful. For example, suppose a client has been avoiding taking steps to organize their personal finances (O1); the therapist and the client have already agreed that avoiding and not asking for help with such tasks is an O1 and the therapist has previously reinforced the client when they asked the therapist (CRB2) what kind of electronic budgeting software they used by telling them the name of the computer program (reinforcer: providing requested tangible support). Now, suppose the client asks the therapist: "Will you share the name of your accountant with me?" Providing the name of the accountant would likely reinforce the client's CRB2 of asking for help and support their O2 of approaching an important avoided task; however, the therapist must be mindful that a multiple relationship would come into being. Depending on the client's particular case conceptualization and the therapist's own personal limits, in some cases it might be advisable to supply the name of the accountant, whereas in others it might be best to support the client in finding alternative strategies for identifying an accountant (e.g., Who else might they ask for a recommendation?). Either way, it is prudent to discuss the potential implications of the multiple relationship that would be formed. Regardless of the specific outcome of this conversation, whether providing the requested help via self-disclosure or setting a limit with the client, this moment provides a potentially fruitful evoke for shaping client behavior (whether in the setting of asking and receiving or asking and respecting a limit) and protecting the sanctity of the therapeutic relationship.

Multiple relationships may also be an important consideration in the provision of supervision and consultation in FAP. Given the deeply interpersonal nature of this work, and the use of the clinician's own warm presence as the primary tool, the content covered in a supervisory relationship is much more likely to include one's personal history or private life than may arise in other forms of CBT consultation or supervision. A helpful question for the supervisor-supervisee dyad to use as a guide is, "Are we exploring an issue in personal life that affects the therapist's skill and emotional availability as a therapist?" Explicitly inviting this question into the room, and considering when the answer is in the affirmative, can reinforce disclosure by the supervisee with confidence that their supervisor is mindful and respectful of the nature of the relationship.

FAP and working with love ethically

In FAP, real and authentic feelings between client and therapist are essential aspects of the therapy. Just as the therapist might feel bored, angry, or pushed away by the client, and might amplify those feelings in the service of shaping more effective interpersonal behavior, so too, both client and therapist may feel loving feelings toward one another.

When the client feels love for the therapist, and expresses that, we would want to consider the function of such an expression. If the expression is a CRB1, that is, the therapist feels uncomfortable, frightened, or pushed away, and if the client has experienced such reactions in their daily life, then the therapist would want to shape more effective forms of the client expressing loving feelings. If the client expresses loving feelings, and historically this has been avoided or hidden in daily life, and the therapist feels warm, inviting, and tender, the therapist would want to honor such feelings, as the client would be engaging in a CRB2. Honoring might involve taking the emotional expression seriously, deeply acknowledging the feelings, identifying the function of them, and helping the client to discriminate contexts in which those feelings can be reciprocated in a balanced way. It is worthy to clarify that therapists are prohibited from engaging in romantic expressions of love (e.g., flirting, kissing, etc.) toward a client, and none of these are considered appropriate behaviors in FAP, as it is hard to imagine these behaviors ever actually helping the client, no matter how persuasive or evocative the client's behavior may be!

It can occur that not only might the client express feelings of love for the therapist, but also may wish for more, such as romance and/or friendship outside of therapy. These feelings and wants, from a FAP perspective, may be very real, genuine, and understandable yearnings that any person would have for another when the relationship is intense and meaningful. A skillful therapist can learn to honor these feelings while carefully reiterating the boundaries of therapy, that therapy is both a personal (real) relationship, while at the same time being a professional relationship that will not evolve into friendship or romance outside of the session. Understandably, the client may feel very sad or even angry about the limitations of the relationship. Learning to feel heartbreak about the limitations of a therapy relationship is an important part of how to love, both in and out of session. Children, for example, learn that while they may love their parents, they will not marry them or have sex with them. This can be painful for the child. Adults, when we love one another, must learn to accept the existential reality that no relationship lasts forever. Death and other goodbyes can be painful, yet they do not have to diminish the reality and depth of love occurring in the present. Learning to love while accepting unwanted and painful boundaries and limitations is an essential part of having close and loving relationships.

The therapist may also feel loving feelings for their client, in fact, we believe that this happens often in FAP due to the emotional and human connection that the therapy promotes. FAP therapists must be very self-aware and have good consultation if those feelings grow and a boundary violation feels tempting. A FAP therapist is bound and supported by the guidelines for ethical behavior for psychologists and other mental health practitioners. FAP therapists must always be guided by what is beneficial for the client, not for themselves, and the power differential in therapy, along with ethical guidelines, would warn against ever violating the boundaries of the therapist/client relationship, as well as that of the supervisor/supervisee relationship. This is both hard and meaningful, as both client and therapist can grow from feeling deeply and not diminishing those feelings because of the boundaries.

15

Diversity, privilege, power, and justice in FAP

As may have become clear at this stage of the book, embracing one's role as a FAP therapist and the primary "tool" in the therapy room requires a high standard of cultural humility, cultural curiosity, and an awareness of one's own privilege and power in the therapy room.

There is an inherent power differential in a therapeutic relationship. We know more about the client than they do about us, ordinarily they pay us for services, and while we then benefit financially from the relationship, we also are working for the client, and they are the consumers of our services. We are viewed as "experts," and thus our overt and implicit bias can be very impactful, a force for good as well as a force that is oppressive and cruel. The inherent power differential in the therapeutic relationship can be a strong evoke for life histories where the power differential has been harmful to the client.

It is worth noting that in many contexts in the United States, where most of the authors of this book are writing, there is a taboo against openly discussing visible differences according to race or cultural differences. This is referred to as *color-blind racial ideology* and may accompany beliefs that avoiding the acknowledgment of difference is a superior means of promoting equality and comfort (Neville et al., 2013). Such avoidance of discussing differences, particularly in regard to visibly recognizable ethnic and racial differences, functions in an opposite manner depending on if one belongs to a majority or minoritized group. For White, culturally powerful individuals, particularly therapists, not acknowledging difference can reduce discomfort with the prospect of discussing racism and injustice. For a Black client in therapy, a therapist's avoidance may function to heighten uncertainty that the therapist would be willing to discuss distressing racist experiences or traumas.

A FAP therapist should be aware of the stimulus value, first and foremost, of their embodied appearance in the room. Regardless of ancestry, are they perceived as White or typically racialized in some way? Regardless of gender identity, are they perceived as a man or woman, as gender conforming, and how do such perceptions affect clients upon a first encounter? It is also important to note how deeply intersectional such identities are, and how the topography of power and privilege may shift as identities are disclosed or discovered over the course of therapy. In a longer course of therapy, the natural process of aging and the inherently temporary nature of able-bodiedness may lead to shifts in the relative power within a dyad of a therapist and client over time.

Holding deep compassion and care for one's client and their experience of the world naturally align with a commitment toward social justice and a desire that each client might have the greatest ability to pursue a life of meaning and connection. Doing so requires that a FAP therapist reflect on those identities that are most privileged and apply effort toward understanding those different from them. Does your social life involve close or meaningful friends of different races, cultures, genders, and sexual orientations? Have you experienced meaningful connections with individuals who differ in body size and shape, nation of origin, or wealth background? Seeking out opportunities to share cultural experiences should not be done with an expectation of complete understanding, it is rather with the humble goal of cultivating cultural appreciation. Ultimately, our clients and their own desires and hopes for connection and vulnerability will determine how a functional analysis incorporates cultural differences in treatment.

That FAP therapists are tuned into "what is the function" of any and all behavior, can promote seeing every client in a way that is unique to them and can minimize therapeutic bias. Understanding the function of behavior is impossible without considering our cultures and meaningful identities. While not deterministic, an awareness of these factors might be helpful in developing hypotheses about what a client's CRB1s or CRB2s are (e.g., Hayes & Toarmino, 1995). Further, the clinician should be aware of their own T1s and T2s in response to those with different identities than their own. A person of color who is seeing a White therapist will bring with them their whole history with White people, and especially their history of asking for help from a White therapist. The therapist, as well, brings with them their entire history with people of color. How would the FAP therapist know how to respond to this? Unlike some approaches that might have a cookie-cutter way to address this kind of disparity, the FAP therapist would want to first be aware that there may be meaningful history informing the interaction. The therapist who is "blind" to the possibility that past harms may be present at the moment would be missing meaningful opportunities in the session and would be violating Rule one, that is to be aware. It is also possible to inquire directly about the life history that would inform this new relationship. How do you feel about starting therapy with me, a White person? Further, the clinician should be aware of their own T1s and T2s in response to those with different identities than their own. In the United States, for example, an initial hypothesis might be that a person of color might have experienced T1s by past therapists in response to the CRB2 of vulnerably disclosing racial microaggressions and their impact during a therapy session, or that a queer client describing challenges in relationships or dating that express vulnerable CRB2s were similarly responded to with T1s based on a therapist's discomfort with the topics. Clients might have trepidation due to their history, a positive mindset due to their history, or difficulty describing their feelings or they also might have sufficiently positive life histories that the question is not relevant, and they want to jump right into the reason for the appointment.

FAP, as an analytic framework, would promote sensitivity to whatever history the client was bringing in with them. Thus, there is no particular way of working with the topics of this chapter with FAP, as the entire analytic framework is based on idiographic, functional analysis. Of course, this is done through the therapist's particular lens, which is itself born of our culture which is riddled with our own history and bias. However, having humility, good supervision, and doing a good functional analysis would sensitize the therapist to these implicit areas of bias and hopefully would help illuminate nonconscious ways of diminishing someone's pain when it is different from ours (Miller et al., 2015).

Using FAP to improve awareness and connection in racially diverse client-therapist dyads

These contexts all point to the importance and centrality of curiosity, openness, respect, and self-education on the part of the FAP clinician. FAP therapists often use questions or therapeutic tasks in order to evoke a CRB2. In this way, anti-racist and social justice oriented FAP therapists might explicitly note, "What is this experience like of sitting here with me as a White therapist, as a Black person with your own history and experiences? Do you have any fears or concerns?" Such evocative statements come with a caveat, however. While the burden of responding to bids for closeness and vulnerability with a T2 is on the therapist, it may not necessarily be a CRB2 for a client to disclose their experiences as a minoritized person with the therapist. The cultural learning history of most majority group therapists in individualistic cultures such as the United States might also predispose a clinician to wait for a client to broach the topic if they deem it meaningful, while the learning history of those with minoritized identities may suggest that a majority-group therapist who does not introduce the topic of obvious differences is likely uncomfortable with it. For these reasons, a majority group FAP therapist should assume that it would be ideally evocative for promoting a vulnerable relationship to introduce the topic of difference first. This does not mean that a FAP therapist does not defer to a client's assertion of boundaries around whether or not they wish to explore their experiences of difference in the therapy room. The goal of FAP therapy is, after all, that the client experiences a sense of thriving amidst meaningful, intimate connections in their life with discrimination of which relationships they most wish to explore those themes within, not that their relationship with their therapist entitles the therapist to cross boundaries.

When a client comes to a FAP therapist for help, we aspire to provide a therapy that is client-centered, respectful of the client's history and longings, and ensure that the work that we do together with the client is respectful and affirming of what is going to help the client live a life that is meaningful to them. The life histories of both client and therapist interact and we believe FAP offers a framework for understanding the function of behavior that encompasses the life history and dynamics of both the client and the therapist.

FAP transcends the notion of topographical categories and getting things right, and instead embraces a functional analytic approach to knowing and understanding a person. For example, one author of this chapter is Jewish, and when wished "Happy Hanukkah" during the holidays, I appreciate the effort made in the sense of not assuming I am part of the majority culture. However, a more meaningful question would be "how is this time of year for you?" A question that invites a more vulnerable response, one that would reflect an actual description of a history of this time being joyful, a feeling of not belonging, grief, awkwardness, and so on. The other author of this chapter, a queer man, has noted the way in which discussion of LGBTQ+ clients is often singled out, creating an unvoiced assumption that clients whose sexual orientation or gender identity are not stated are cisgender and heterosexual. For this reason, he began noting in consultation and professional discussions any of a client's identities, leading a FAP colleague to ask if this indicated that the author had a particular fixation on heterosexual or cisgender identities. While such a microaggression—in this case, interpersonally punishing the violation of a rule that treats cisgender and heterosexual identities as an unspoken norm that reflects unself-conscious cis-heterocentrism—a better question might have been, "I notice you label when clients are heterosexual, and I usually do not. What is this practice in the service of?" FAP invites vulnerability, getting it wrong, getting it right, and working toward a deeper connection.

Part II

THE DISTINCTIVE PRACTICAL FEATURES OF FAP

This section encompasses all the practical and experiential dimensions of FAP. It provides a detailed description of FAP's functional assessment and treatment procedures, illustrating how these can be implemented across various settings and integrated with other therapeutic approaches.

DOI: 10.4324/9781032694832-17

16

Setting the stage: Creating a sacred space of trust and safety

The importance of fostering trust and safety cannot be overstated in FAP. The therapist may choose to describe this process as "creating a sacred space" for therapeutic work. According to the *Oxford Dictionary*, a sacred space is dedicated, set apart, exclusively appropriated to some person or special purpose, and is protected by sanction from injury or incursion. Use of this term with clients may be quite powerful. Whether or not a FAP therapist chooses to use the term "sacred space" with clients, the key issue is that, functionally, the relationship is indeed sacred as defined here, and creating trust and safety is essential (Tsai et al., 2019).

For the typical FAP client, however, fostering trust and safety may move beyond these basic therapy skills and into areas that are much more personal and genuine. Therapists can foster a sense of trust and safety with these clients by being more forthcoming with their thoughts, reactions, and observations (not hiding behind a therapist persona). And they can encourage clients: (a) to ask questions (e.g., "What are your questions about me, my training, my background?" or "What qualities do you most seek in a therapist?"); (b) to voice their reactions to the therapist (e.g., "What reactions do you have to my gender, age, ethnicity?"); and (c) to voice their feelings related to the appointment (e.g., "What are your thoughts and feelings about having this appointment today?" or "What would make this a really good first session for you?"). The FAP therapist, however, remains open to the possibility that some therapist behaviors may be aversive to specific clients depending on their histories, so assessment of the therapist's stimulus functions is important from the very beginning of therapy.

Numerous behaviors can help to engender another's trust. These trust-building behaviors are not specific to the therapy situation. In FAP, we do not believe the therapist becomes a different person when stepping into a therapy room. Rather, behaviors that are well practiced and integrated outside therapy are more likely to succeed in the therapy room. These trust-enhancing behaviors may include: (a) providing accurate empathic reflections; (b) being honest and genuine; (c) keeping one's word; (d) being consistent and predictable, or explaining why one is being inconsistent and unpredictable so that the behavior makes sense; (e) recognizing another's expectations, and correcting them if not accurate, or explaining why one is not meeting them; (f) admitting when one does not know the answer; (g) seeing what is in someone's best interest and not taking advantage of or hurting him or her; (h) remembering the important things someone has revealed—people, events, memories; (i) being willing to match the other person's vulnerability; (j) being able to admit and take responsibility for mistakes, to repair ruptures; and (k) treating client truths and disclosures with care and reverence.

Trust, behaviorally speaking, may be seen as a predisposition to approach another person in a situation in which one could potentially get hurt. Thus, trust essentially describes a situation in which one person is predisposed to take risks in the presence of, and toward, another person. Instilling trust and safety are crucial in FAP because clients are shaped and reinforced to take risks, to be vulnerable, to push beyond their boundaries of comfort, and to take more steps to trust the therapist. That said, the behavior of trusting may be a goal of therapy and it is the rare client who will trust fully from the first session. Indeed, such blind trust may be as problematic as an inability to trust.

Fostering a sense of trust and safety, as everything else in FAP, is an idiographic process. Thus, for many clients, a host of what has been referred to as "nonspecific" behaviors, such as accurate empathy, warmth, reflective listening, and validation, may be very important early therapist behaviors toward this end.

Although many theorists, particularly Carl Rogers (1961), argue that the important quality of such nonspecific therapist responses is that they are unconditional (not contingent on particular client responses), the FAP therapist takes a different stance. As described more fully by Follette, Naugle, and Callaghan (1996), the FAP therapist's responses are seen as potentially reinforcing broad classes of behaviors (e.g., trusting and other therapy-facilitating and relationship-building behaviors). The therapist's behaviors are seen as generalized contingent reinforcement for the class of behaviors necessary for therapy to occur and a relationship to develop. This class includes behaviors like trusting, showing up on time, disclosing important personal information, paying attention and responding appropriately to questions, demonstrating caring and concern for the therapist's feelings, and being engaged in session.

In the service of client growth, we not only shape our clients' behavior, but allow ourselves in turn to be shaped by our clients. As Martin Buber (n.d.) stated, "All journeys have secret destinations of which the traveler is unaware." Allow yourself to experience each therapeutic relationship as within a sacred space on such a journey.

17

Functional analysis and case conceptualization in FAP

Many therapists may start treatment focused on diagnostic assessment. Such an assessment can be helpful and may lead the therapist to choose specific empirically based treatment (EBT) strategies to administer. For example, a clinician may choose to conduct ACT (Hayes et al., 1999), Cognitive Therapy (Beck et al., 1979), or Behavioral Activation (Martell et al., 2010) for a client presenting "depressive symptomatology", following the EBT recommendations. On the contrary, FAP therapists are focused on the function of behavior (see Chapter 3); therefore, treatment selection is preceded by a case conceptualization that unveiled the function of the problem and its learning history.

Whether in the context of another treatment or not, FAP case conceptualization moves beyond diagnostic assessment and focuses on idiographically identifying and defining CRBs in such a way that maximizes the possibility that the therapist will observe, evoke, and reinforce them in session. The therapist's goal is to understand the client's interpersonal behavioral repertoires—how they function in the client's daily life, and how they function in the therapy room. There is no correct way to do this in FAP, but in general we distinguish between attempts to assess in-session behaviors and out-of-session behaviors.

The starting point for case conceptualization in FAP is functional analysis (FA), a methodology developed in the early 90's by Brian Iwata, a renowned behavior analyst (Hanley et al., 2003). Behavior analysts developed three types of functional analysis (Cooper et al., 2020):

1. Experimental: examine behavior's functions through arranging analog situations to systematically test various conditions (antecedents and consequences).
2. Descriptive: directly observe the natural occurrence of behavior in context to identify the relations between antecedents, responses, and consequences.

DOI: 10.4324/9781032694832-19

3. Indirect: organize information from multimethod (e.g., self-records, instruments) and multi sources (e.g., clients, caregivers) to determine behavior's functions with no direct observations of the behaviors and environment.

FA allows collecting and organizing information in the present moment, identifying current contingencies controlling the behavior but not past contingencies. Most assessments in clinical settings with verbally and cognitively able individuals are based on indirect functional analysis as direct observations or manipulation of context are unfeasible. Nonetheless, the relational nature of FAP made it viable to employ both descriptive and indirect FA in order to identify whether the function of client's interpersonal behaviors outside of session are similar to those in-session. First, therapists can utilize self-records and scales to determine the function of client's interpersonal problems in their daily life (Outside Problems-OI) using an indirect FA. Second, they can use a descriptive FA to observe the natural flow of contingencies in the therapeutic session (Rule 1) to determine what is controlling client's interpersonal difficulties in-session (CRBIs). Aftermath, therapists can merge the information from both indirect and descriptive FA to identify the common contextual sources that control OIs and CRBIs.

Whatever the method, the important issue is that the FAP therapist is trying to identify clinically relevant interpersonal operant behaviors that occur both in the client's daily life and in the therapy room. It is essential that these behaviors are defined as *functional classes* or sets of behaviors that are defined by similar antecedents and consequences, rather than by similar forms. For example, a quintessential CRB1 in FAP is avoidance of genuine intimate expression. To understand this as a functional class, we would seek to understand what sorts of contexts trigger the behavior and what sorts of consequences follow it. Essentially, when faced with the opportunity to express genuine intimacy, the client escapes or avoids the situation, thereby avoiding feared negative consequences. This avoidance may look very different from situation to situation. In a family context, it may take the form of literal flight, while in therapy, the client may stay in the situation but make jokes or express hostility. All of these behaviors would be considered in the same functional class in FAP.

A FAP case conceptualization form that is used by many FAP therapists to merge indirect and descriptive FAs includes the following categories (see Table 17.1, inspired by Tsai et al., 2009): relevant history, O1s (Functional classes of daily life problems), CRB1s, CRB2s, O2s (Functional classes of daily life goals), assets and strengths, planned interventions, T1s (therapist in-session problems) and T2 (therapist in-session target behaviors). In this case conceptualization, the relevant history section includes information from past contingencies as well as cultural practices that contribute to O1s and CRB1s origin and maintenance. While past contingencies cannot be modified, they are key to understanding how client's behaviors developed and how pervasive

Table 17.1 *Functional Analytic Psychotherapy Case Conceptualization*

Relevant history	Historical factors contributing to the development of O1s, encompassing biological, cultural, or social events of relevance.
O1s (Functional classes of daily life problems)	Group of responses maintained by similar consequences (i.e., positive or negative reinforcement). This section delves into problematic behaviors and their controlling contextual factors, including contextual cues, consequences, rules, and more.
CRB1	Client's in-session responses that meet the same function as O1s.
CRB2s	Client's improvements in sessions that involve alternative repertoire to CRB1s. These behavioral repertoires enhance the access to positive natural reinforcement.
O2s (Functional classes of daily life goals)	Group of responses maintained by the same consequences. It includes a description of the alternative behaviors and controlling contextual factors such as contextual cues, consequences, rules, among others.
Assets and strengths	Client's skills and contextual strengths that could support behavioral change and maintenance of progress.
Planned interventions	Therapeutic procedures intended for implementation, which have shown effectiveness in targeting the antecedents, behaviors, or consequences associated with O1s and CRB1s, as well as positively influencing O2s and CRB2s.
T1s (therapist in-session problems)	Therapist's interpersonal difficulties that could interfere with treatment implementation or the client's progress.
T2 (therapist in-session target behaviors)	Therapist's interpersonal strengths that can enhance treatment implementation or the client's progress.

they are. In addition, clients' assets and strengths are identified in order to acknowledge protective factors that can be utilized to aid the client to thrive through the therapeutic process. Finally, therapists' interpersonal problems (T1s) and strengths (T2) are described to acknowledge the interpersonal nature of FAP in which therapists' difficulties, as the contexts in session, can hinder the client's progress, and therapist's strengths support it, and as so, therapist need to be aware of their own limitations and skills to prevent any interference and take the maximum advantage of their strengths in-session, respectively.

18

The treatment rationale and the beginning of therapy

The therapy rationale is a discussion that takes place with clients at the beginning of treatment. It offers an explanation of the possible causes of the presenting problems (case conceptualization; see Chapter 17) as well as a description of what the treatment will be like. The rationale is important because it helps to set the context for the types of intervention used in FAP and moderates therapeutic alliance issues that can be brought about by disparate expectations between client and therapist. For this reason, we recommend formally presenting a rationale, whether written or verbal. If such a statement is not made, the client draws on experience or common knowledge about what any treatment will entail, and if that picture is different from the therapist's plan, it may impede progress.

Other than affirming that the therapist-client relationship is both a focus and a key factor in achieving treatment goals, there is no one-size-fits-all FAP rationale (also known as FAP Rapport—"FAP Rap"). The examples below contain a range of FAP rationales that illustrate: (a) ways therapists may adapt their rationales to fit their therapy approaches, (b) therapy parameters (e.g., brief or longer-term), (c) treatment goals, and (d) the amount of risk taken by the therapist in terms of how evocative the rationale is. Frequently, even mentioning that there will be a focus on the therapist-client relationship might be evocative of CRB.

Example 1: Rationale given in the second therapy session

The following stated rationale and the client's reaction to it took place during the second treatment session. In the first session, the client reported that her primary problems included unhappiness, low self-esteem, a sense that she was not a good person, and the belief that others, especially her mother, generally thought poorly of her. During the

 DOI: 10.4324/9781032694832-20

second session, the therapist focused on how she perceived his feelings and reactions to her and then presented the following:

> *T:* You'll notice I've talked a lot about the two of us, and I want to tell you why. I think that one of the most powerful ways for therapy to be effective is to actually work on your problems as they are occurring, so, for example, if you're upset about your mother or having difficulty relating to your mother, we might sit here and talk about it. That might be helpful. We can figure out how you feel and how she feels and so on, and we'll do some of that. But it's more powerful if the problems you're having you actually experience in the relationship with me. So, for example, you did. That is, you reacted to what happened at the end of the last session very much in the same way that's modeled after your reaction to Mom.
>
> *C:* Right.
>
> *T:* The therapy is just more powerful and effective if you can actually grasp on these things while they're occurring. So, I wanted to let you know why I've been asking you these questions and focusing on our relationship.

Example 2: Excerpt from a highly evocative written rationale

Clients come into therapy with complex life stories of joy and anguish, dreams and hopes, passions and vulnerabilities, unique gifts and abilities. Your therapy with me will be conducted in an atmosphere of caring, respect and commitment in which new ways of approaching life are learned. Our work will be a joint effort; your input is valued and will be used in the treatment plan and in weekly homework assignments. I will be investing a great deal of care and effort into our work together, and I expect you to do the same. I will be checking with you in an ongoing way about what is working well for you in our relationship and what needs to be changed.

The type of therapy that I will be doing is called Functional Analytic Psychotherapy (FAP). It is a therapy developed at the University of Washington that is behaviorally based but has the theoretical foundation to incorporate methods from other therapeutic modalities when appropriate. FAP emphasizes that the bond that will be formed between you and me will be a major vehicle in your healing and transformation.

The most fulfilled people are in touch with themselves and are able to be interpersonally effective. They are able to speak and act compassionately on their truths and gifts and are able to fully give and receive love. FAP will focus on bringing forth your best self. In order to do that, you must first be in touch with yourself at a core level (e.g., needs, feelings, longings, fears, values, dreams, missions). You will have the opportunity to learn how to express yourself fully, to grieve losses, to develop mindfulness, and to create better relationships. All aspects of your experience will be addressed, including mind, body, feelings, and spirit. I will be challenging you to be more open, vulnerable, aware and present. There is an optimal level of risk-taking in any situation, however, and it's important that you and I monitor how much outside your comfort zone is best for you at any given time.

It will be important for us to focus on our interaction if you have issues (positive or negative) or difficulties that come up with me which also come up with other people in your life. When one feels the power in expressing one's thoughts, feelings, and desires in an authentic, caring and assertive way, one has a greater sense of mastery in life. Our therapeutic relationship will be an ideal place for you to practice being powerful.

I consider the space that you enter with me in therapy to be sacred— I am privileged to be embarking on a journey of exploration and growth with you, and I will hold all that you share with reverence and with care. I will be a genuine person in the room with you, and my main guiding principle is to do that which is in your best interest.

Example 3: Excerpt from a less evocative version of the above

FAP often includes the empirically supported Cognitive Behavior Therapy protocols for specific disorders. At the same time, FAP emphasizes that the therapist-client relationship is important for accomplishing significant life change. Thus, in addition to a specific symptom focus as needed, FAP also provides the opportunity to bring forth your best self, to learn how to express yourself fully, to grieve losses as needed, to develop mindfulness, and to create better relationships.

It will be important for us to focus on our interaction if you have issues (positive or negative) or difficulties that come up with me which also come up with other people in your life. Our therapeutic relationship will be an ideal place for you to practice being more effective in your relationships with others.

Example 4: Rationale given in a FAP-informed brief treatment study

> *T:* This study is about helping you to increase feelings of closeness and respect in your relationship. Contrary to a lot of other therapies that focus on telling you how to do things, the way we will try to help you increase your ability to have closeness is to actually practice it between you and me. Research shows that really effective therapists tend to think about how what is showing up here between you and me in the therapy room is showing up in your relationship. For example, for your goal of wanting to be more thoughtful in your relationship, we then ask how can thoughtfulness occur here, between us? How do we know that you're actually working on being a thoughtful person here, in this brand-new relationship with me? That's the premise of this sort of work and what we will be dealing with.
>
> *C:* So, if I may ask, is the idea that this is a study to try to validate that enacting some of the behavioral changes here that we're wanting to manifest in the primary relationship can happen more readily if you practice it specifically in our therapeutic relationship?
>
> *T:* Yes, and it's not role-playing. It's actually much more powerful when it's real and happening between us, and I can give you really authentic and genuine feedback. For example, you were being thoughtful in the way that you asked about and tried to understand what I was doing. It made me feel more comfortable with you and it sounded like you actually cared.

The above examples illustrate the primary theme present in FAP: a focus on the therapist-client relationship as a real relationship that plays a central role in the change process. In each case, the FAP rationale is the therapist's personal invitation to the client to participate in a meaningful interpersonal relationship.

19

Introduction to the five rules

Doing FAP has generally been presented as a dance among five thera-peutic rules that describe the ways in which the therapist orients their attention toward the client and engages in flexible perspective-taking and tacting of felt sensations. The term "rule" might falsely give the impression of rigidity. These are not rules in the sense of command-ments, rather an organizing structure that, when followed, increases the likelihood that both the client and the therapist will be shaped into a direction of more workable interpersonal behaviors. These rules might guide therapists in taking advantage of therapeutic opportunities that may otherwise go unnoticed (Tsai et al., 2009).

While the five rules are described in the language of operant con-ditioning, FAP also acknowledges the presence of respondent, or classical, conditioning in our learning histories. Frequent pairings of markers of gender, race, sexual orientation, or able-bodiedness all cor-respond to sensory cues that have been associated throughout a cli-ent's life with danger or safety, kindness or judgment. The behaviors targeted in therapy arise within that specific context, sensitive to these prior types of learning. Our cultures shape and reinforce the manner in which we express our emotions, both verbally and non-verbally. Though not emphasized within the rules, a FAP clinician should con-sider such prior learning.

Rule 1: Notice CRBs (be aware)

The first half of this volume emphasized paying attention to the func-tion of behavior because, without the ability to see behaviors as func-tional units, a therapist will be unable to determine what CRBs arise in the room. It is through the focus on those behaviors that arise in the room, rather than questions about behavior in the world, that allow FAP to delve so deeply into interpersonal processes. Determining how

DOI: 10.4324/9781032694832-21

problems in life manifest within relationships increases the likelihood of powerful change as a result of the therapy.

Rule 2: Evoke CRBs (be courageous)

Two considerations must be made prior to evoking CRBs in the room. First, clients may have prior histories with psychotherapy that emphasized the content of their words and the reporting of behaviors that occurred outside of therapy. This may initially block the natural expression of CRBs within the therapeutic relationship. Second, the therapist must fully express themselves as a person, not a "blank slate," in order to hold evocative potential. An adage that the second author (MDS) was fond of reminding his students was to "keep it awkward." That is, when therapy seems overly smooth, comfortable, yet lacking in substance, the therapist might consider how their own behavior has failed to evoke meaningful responses from the client. The therapist might consider if the energy that they bring into the room should be higher, lower, or if their range of emotional expression is weaker than the client is responsive to. The therapist must become acquainted with taking courageous risks to truly present as a whole person, authentically disclosing emotional responses to the client's experiences, and bringing a natural and warm curiosity to the therapeutic encounter.

Rule 3: Effectively consequating CRBs— naturally (be therapeutically loving)

It is unlikely that a client participates in the therapeutic relationship with only CRB1s at the start. Many clients may express CRB2s that are under-rehearsed, inconsistently evoked, or respond to stimuli such as internal rules about behavior with strangers that may weaken over time as the therapy progresses. This may lead to the assumption that Rule 3 encourages reinforcement as the primary instrument of change, though unnatural reinforcement can become contrived, and the same behavioral principles that FAP is built upon suggest that a continuous schedule of reinforcement (i.e., reinforcing a behavior every time it occurs) leads to a low rate of change and low effort. Such styles of reinforcement or schedules of reinforcement that are too frequent can also be experienced as aversive or manipulative by the client. Natural reinforcers are those styles of responses within the behavioral repertoire of an individual therapist that express their own unique manner of relating.

In FAP, this is sometimes referred to as therapeutic loving, and while not all therapists are comfortable with using the word *love* in (Muñoz-Martínez & Follette, 2019) reference to the behavior of a therapist (and the processes of shaping, reinforcing, and blocking), it is important that the therapist has their own learning history and perspective-taking behaviors established enough to respond with warmth. To be therapeutically loving is, within the boundaries of ethics and professionalism, to commit to that natural wellspring of warmth that the therapist draws upon within their own life and relationships. As elaborated in Chapter 22, the FAP therapist might consider this rule to be one of responsiveness. The therapeutic space is one in which the therapist pays warm, close attention to the behavior of the client and responds in a manner that is both naturally caring enough to reinforce the behavior while amplified to a degree that it orients the client to their impact on the therapist.

Rule 4: Observe the potentially reinforcing effects of therapist behavior in relation to CRBs (be aware of one's impact)

Much like CRBs, therapist responses are also defined functionally. That is, a behavior is not reinforcing because it feels good to the therapist, or because other clients have responded in the expected manner. Rule 4 calls attention to the importance of noting whether a specific therapist's behavior, in response to a specific CRB2, leads to an increase in the frequency of that CRB2. Only then can we be certain that the client is reinforced by the therapist in a predictable manner. It is equally important for the therapist to consider their contingent responding in the presence of CRB1s that appear to have maintained or increased their frequency. One CRB1 that many therapists find challenging, for example, is laughter when it is used to stifle or block an avoided emotion such as sadness, fear, or shame. As social animals, most people have been raised in environments where one person's laughter evokes their own, and it feels good to laugh, as an added source of reinforcement! Laughing along with our client's self-deprecatory humor that blocks the experience of sadness, however, only increases that CRB1. The FAP therapist will notice this and attempt to respond in a different way. They might introduce the topic early in a session and share a sign or gesture they will use to point out when they believe the client is engaging in this behavior, or they might sit with a still face until the laughter subsides and ask the client what feeling was present that did not have to be felt as a result of the laughter.

When effective, a therapist might ask how it felt to be responded to in this manner. Perhaps they were moved by a client's disclosure of pain, and the client's own history was full of important figures who neglected the client. While explicit questions, such as "What was it like for you when you noticed the tears in my eyes and I shared how moved I was by your story?" may be helpful for the therapist in determining the function of their behavior, such questions should not follow too closely to the reinforcing behavior. This risks undermining the emotional impact of the interaction that occurred immediately prior. In waiting for the ebb of strong emotions that may have been evoked in the meeting of a CRB2 with a natural reinforcer, such questions might need to occur in a subsequent session.

Rule 5: Provide functional analytically informed interpretations and implement generalization strategies (interpret and generalize)

Interpretations in a functional analytically informed therapy are not the same as those stereotypically offered in a psychodynamic or psychoanalytic approach. The goal of a functional analytic interpretation is to offer a model to the client that describes how their own learning history, and those behaviors that were reinforced by their environment and the people around them, resulted in those behaviors that are now experienced as problems. These might be "out-to-in parallels" that describe how behavior patterns that occur in daily life are arising within the therapeutic encounter, or they might be "in-to-out parallels" when an in-session improvement corresponds to a similarly successful change in daily life. Both are important, and FAP sessions typically involve the incorporation of both.

Further, a key aspect of generalizing new skills is in the act of discrimination. That is, a successful outcome in FAP is not that a person responds universally with vulnerable disclosures or aspires to create intimacy in every relationship, but rather that one attends to the stimuli presented and orients externally to moment-by-moment feedback presented by another person in place of orienting internally toward verbal rules about how to build a relationship. Following a meaningful exchange, the therapist might ask a client, "What was it about me that helped this feel like a safe moment to share this part of yourself? Who else in your life do you notice those qualities in?" Such evocative statements might help shape a repertoire of discriminating antecedent contingencies, though the same shaping might occur by noting responses from others. That is, the client might be encouraged to consider what felt most meaningful in the therapist's response (following the practice of Rule 4), and then to consider what types of responses would suggest that another person is responding in a manner that encourages further vulnerable disclosures. In this way, the client might be encouraged to consider how consequatingconsequating contingencies might signal another's willingness or desire to deepen a relationship.

The goal of FAP is ultimately to improve daily life, not to create a more pleasurable therapeutic experience. To that end, successful new behaviors in therapy might lead to an in-to-out reflection and the collaborative development of homework that might expose the client to natural reinforcement by meaningful others in their life. For example, a client who discloses a painful life event that moves the therapist deeply, yielding a sense of deeper connection between therapist and client, might be encouraged to disclose this major life event to someone meaningful in everyday life with whom they hope to experience greater intimacy or vulnerability.

20

Observing (Rule 1)

When a client comes in for any variety of therapy, the therapist must grow awareness of the client's struggles and their strengths. This awareness is key to setting the stage for intense, interpersonally focused, and effective therapy. Rule 1, in FAP, captures this imperative. Rule 1 states that the therapist "is aware of the client's clinically relevant behaviors (CRBs), as they occur, in session." Rule 1, awareness, is critical to better, more accurate detection of and then therapeutic responses to CRBs. Without the therapist being aware of the client's suffering and their longings and gifts, a client would rightfully feel unseen and misunderstood, which would likely sabotage the therapeutic experience. Awareness, the ability to notice our clients, the ability to notice our world, is the first step in growing connection and thus the ability to engage and move in valued directions. Finding our way in total darkness is next to impossible; light, observing, or awareness is required to be in contact with the humans in our presence as well as the physicality and contingencies of our world. Therapists can sharpen their ability to detect CRBs in several ways, some of which are described below.

Be aware of therapeutic situations that frequently evoke CRBs

Situations that often evoke CRBs include time structure (i.e., 45–50-minute hour), fees, and/or therapist characteristics (e.g., age, gender, race, attractiveness, office setting, either in person or online). CRBs may be evoked by a silence in the conversation, a client's expression of affect, a client doing well, a therapist providing positive feedback or expressions of caring, and/or a client feeling close to the therapist. Still others could be a therapist's vacations, mistakes, personal distractions, or unintentional behavior; unusual events such as a client seeing the therapist with a partner outside of therapy or seeing something personal in an session if the therapist is working from home, the therapist becoming pregnant, the therapist becoming ill or wearing a wedding ring (or taking one off), and/or therapy termination. Evokes can also be such things as starting therapy after having ended therapy with a beloved or hated therapist. CRBs associated with grief or self-protection could be seen very early in the therapy. When circumstances like these occur, being aware of possible CRBs and probing for client reactions can lead to more productive therapy.

Use your own reactions as data

A therapist's personal reactions to a client can be a valuable sensor for CRBs. Generally, how we feel toward our clients may be similar to how others in their life feel about them. Questions you can ask yourself include: What are the ways your client pushes you away emotionally? Does your attention wander because s/he talks tangentially or avoids eye contact? Is s/he avoidant of your questions? Does s/he frustrate you because they take none of your suggestions, or take all of them and not do them, or be perfectionistic? Does s/he say one thing and do another? Is s/he critical of your every intervention? Does s/he pull away when the two of you have had a close interaction? Does s/he seem to have no interest or curiosity in you as a person? A key issue is knowing when your responses to a client are representative of how others in the client's life might respond, and when your responses are idiosyncratic. To the degree your responses are representative, they are a good indicator that CRB may be occurring.

Identify possible CRBs based on FIAT (Functional Idiographic Assessment Template) responses (Callaghan, 2006)

The FIAT is an assessment instrument that identifies five response classes that are associated with interpersonal effectiveness. Darrow et al. (2014) validated a 111-item questionnaire (FIAT-Q) and a 32-item short form (FIAT-Q-SF) that allow identifying these functional classes in a self-reported fashion. Whether or not you use this assessment instrument, we explore the five groups of responses as they are useful in becoming sensitive to client relationship effectiveness.

Class A: Assertion of needs
(identification and expression)

The term "needs" stands for anything that one wants or values. This is important because, in relationships, the ability to state who one is, and what one longs for, is passionate about, and suffers about, is critical to having a close relationship. Imagine a relationship where people stuck to very superficial topics: "I like the color green… cool, I like the color red." And now imagine a relationship where people say: "I am nervous about being here… I am too, I barely slept last night I was so nervous about meeting you…" In session, possible CRB1s include difficulty identifying or expressing what one needs from the therapist. Struggling to express reactions, positive or negative, about the therapist, could be CRB1s.

Class B: Bi-directional communication
(impact and feedback)

This class of behaviors involves how one gives and responds to feedback, both verbal and nonverbal. Possible CRB1s include difficulty receiving and providing either appreciation or constructive criticism, unreasonable expectations of self or therapist, little awareness of or hypersensitivity to impact on therapist, talking too long or too tangentially without checking impact, being too quiet, holding too much or too little eye contact, and exhibiting body language that does not match verbal content.

Class C: Conflict

Intimate relationships involve having disagreements and conflict. Clients who are conflict avoidant, or who express too much anger or self-blame, or express upset indirectly, can push others away and could be CRB1s.

Class D: Disclosure and interpersonal closeness

Being able to be close to another person involves a level of self-disclosure. Feeling understood by others and understanding others involves being able to talk about one's deep feelings and being able to be open to the feelings of others. Possible CRB1s include having difficulty expressing or receiving closeness and care, being reluctant to self-disclosure or take emotional risks, talking too much about oneself, not listening well, not being aware of the therapist's needs (e.g., going overtime, not giving the therapist the opportunity to talk), and having difficulty trusting.

Class E: Emotional experience and expression

The term "emotional experience" refers to all types of emotions, both negative (e.g., sadness, anxiety, loneliness, anger) and positive (e.g., love, pride, joy, humor). Possible CRB1s include difficulty identifying, feeling, and expressing negative or positive feelings, expressing feelings in an overly intense manner, and avoiding emotional expression and experience.

Use a FAP case conceptualization

FAP case conceptualization involves speculating about how your client's stated problems and goals for therapy may show up in the therapy room and then asking questions and observing your client to confirm or modify those hypotheses over time. The therapist may ask "out-to-in" parallel questions about possible in-session instantiations of out-of-session behavior, as in,

> I understand you struggle a great deal with your partner when they are late, really worrying about their safety, and sometimes over-reacting and pushing them away when they do get home. Today, I was late to our session, and then you seemed rather distant, and I wonder if you felt worried and then pushed me away, the way you do with your partner.

Asking such questions that parallel out-of-session and in-session behavior is a standard tool to help with the identification of possible CRBs.

Increased awareness in session requires a heightened sensitivity and connection to your client. In casual conversation, we can sometimes be distracted, but in FAP, the therapist aspires to be fully focused and completely in the moment with the client to an unusual degree. FAP encourages the therapist to be aware of and connected to the client's history of hurts and successes, losses and gains. FAP encourages deep caring and sensitivity on the part of the therapist. No therapist can be 100% present and tuned in all the time. The therapist can be aware and self-disclosing about this, modeling vulnerability and commitment to the connection even when feeling distracted and pulled away by other matters.

It is important for the therapist to enter the therapy session with honesty and openness to the client and to one's own reactions to and feelings about the client. The therapist's capacity and repertoires, both in and out of session, are "practice", that is, we are working to improve our skills of awareness and compassion in all areas of our lives.

FAP therapists aspires to focus on our own in-session problem behaviors and on our own in-session target behaviors. Self-awareness of these repertoires will enhance our skill with respect to helping shape improvements in our clients. We recommend that therapists set aside time to explore questions such as:

1. What do you tend to avoid addressing with your clients?
2. How does this avoidance impact the work that you do with these clients?
3. What do you tend to avoid dealing with in your life (e.g., tasks, people, memories, needs, feelings, or endings)?
4. How do your daily life avoidances impact the work that you do with your clients?
5. What are the specific T2s you want to develop with each client based on his/her case conceptualization?

The client who enters therapy with complaints of feeling flat and dead inside, and who emerges from therapy feeling joy and pain and everything in between—in session with you, as well as in relationships in their daily lives—is an example of Rule 1, leading to an intense, meaningful, and effective therapeutic experience.

21

Evoking (Rule 2)

Implementing the steps to create an evocative therapeutic relationship often entails therapists taking risks and pushing their own intimacy boundaries. Such risks involve being courageous, venturing, persevering, and withstanding fear of difficulty. Doing FAP well often involves stretching one's limits and going outside of one's comfort zone.

Structuring therapy with the FAP Rationale (the FAP Rap)

From the very first contact, as discussed in Chapter 16, therapists can begin structuring the therapeutic environment to prepare the client for an intense and evocative therapy that focuses on in-vivo interactions, by describing the FAP rationale ("FAP Rap"). In order for FAP to be most effective, it is important that clients understand its premise—that the therapist will be looking for ways that clients' outside life problems show up within the therapy relationship because such an in-vivo focus facilitates the most powerful change. This is an atypical idea regarding therapy as most people think they go into therapy to talk about problems and relationships outside of the therapy. Thus, variations of the FAP Rap are presented in the initial phone contact, in the client's informed consent form, and in the early sessions of treatment until the client understands it thoroughly.

Various examples of the FAP Rap might include:

1. *"I will be attempting to identify ways your daily life problems emerge within our therapy relationship, because such an in-vivo focus facilitates the most powerful change."*
2. *"A primary principle in the type of therapy I do is that our relationship is a microcosm of your outside relationships. So, I will be exploring how you interact with me in a way that is similar to how you interact with other people, what problems*

DOI: 10.4324/9781032694832-23

come up with me that also come up with other people, or what positive behaviors you have with me that you can translate into your relationships with other people."

3. *"One focus of our therapy will be on how you can become a more powerful person, someone who can speak your truth compassionately and go after what you want. The most effective way for you to develop into a more expressive person is to start right here, right now, with me, to tell me what you are thinking, feeling, and needing, even if it feels scary or risky. If you can bring forth your best self with me, then you can transfer those behaviors to other people in your life."*

4. *"Our connection provides an opportunity for you to explore how you are in a relationship, for you to experiment with different ways of relating, and then to take it to your other relationships."*

5. *"Therapy has a greater impact when you talk about your experience in the present moment rather than reporting about things felt during the week. When we look at something that is happening right now, we can experience and understand it more fully and therapeutic change is stronger and more immediate."*

6. Again, a more detailed discussion of this topic, along with examples of how the form of the FAP rap can be tailored to match a range of therapist styles and comfort zones, is given in Chapter 18.

Focusing on FIAT-Q response classes

As discussed in Chapters 8 and 20, some therapists may find it helpful to use the FIAT (Callaghan, 2006a) when assessing CRBs in and out of session. Possible therapist behaviors to evoke CRBs in each of the response classes include:

1. Class A (Assertion of needs): Asking certain kinds of questions. "What do you need from me, from this treatment?", "What would make this a really good session for you?", "How do you feel when I take your needs seriously?", "How did you feel when I said no to your request?"

2. Class B (Bi-directional communication): Giving client appreciation and positive feedback, engaging in exercises where both therapist and client give each other positive feedback, asking for and giving constructive criticism, letting the client know his or her impact, asking for more eye contact, and asking for body language to match verbal expression.
3. Class C (Conflict): Bringing up topics that may potentially cause conflict.
4. Class D (Disclosure and interpersonal closeness): Prompting more client self-disclosure, providing therapist self-disclosure if relevant to increasing closeness with the client, letting the client know what s/he does that blocks closeness and inviting behaviors that increase closeness.
5. Class E (Emotional experience and expression): Prompting more client emotional experience and expression, self-disclosing therapist emotional experience in response to the client, helping client with emotion regulation or containment if overly emotional.

For more detail on ways to evoke CRBs, please refer to pp. 70–83 in Tsai et al. (2009).

Using evocative therapeutic methods

FAP is an integrative therapy and calls for varied therapeutic techniques depending on what will evoke client issues and what will be naturally reinforcing of client target behaviors. What is important is not the theoretical origin of a specific technique but its function with a particular client. To the extent that a technique—any technique—functions to help clients contact and express avoided thoughts and feelings and other CRB1s, and evoke CRB2s that can be naturally reinforced, it is potentially useful to FAP.

Techniques often borrowed from other therapeutic approaches include: free association, timed writing exercises (e.g., writing whatever comes to mind without censoring), empty chair work, evoking emotion by focusing on bodily sensations, and evoking a client's best self using visualization. Such techniques are viewed functionally. That is, emotional expressions (e.g., grief or a remembered trauma) are not described as a "release of energy" or "getting out repressed feelings," but rather the expression is considered a CRB2, related to being more open, that will build and strengthen interpersonal closeness.

The general point is that almost any technique can be borrowed from other approaches if employed functionally and used to evoke CRBs. FAP therapists do not need to look like behavior therapists. They need to act like behavior therapists, which means being willing to try techniques that traditionally have not been labeled "behavioral" but doing so in a way that clarifies and uses their functions. In this way, the FAP therapist practices a technical eclecticism in the service of evoking CRBs that never loses its functional, behavioral foundation. Some behavior therapists may be reluctant to stray from specific techniques that they have been taught are the right "behavioral" techniques. We find this to be unnecessarily limiting. It greatly restricts the potential power of FAP. We encourage therapists to challenge themselves in this regard by exploring new techniques with a "try it and see" attitude, while always looking at the function, not the form, of techniques employed (Nelson et al., 2016).

22

Reinforcing/consequating (Rule 3)

Rule 3 entails the strategic use of genuine therapist responses in service of reinforcing client target behaviors (CRB2) and decreasing problematic client behaviors (CRB1s). As psychotherapists, and specifically as FAP therapists, our fundamental commitment to clients is to co-create a therapeutic environment that centers and promotes the client's well-being. In FAP, we refer to this stance and pledge as therapeutic love, though, as contextual behaviorists, we do not mandate that therapists use this specific language (or any other) if it is not befitting them or their clients. To be therapeutically loving/responsive requires that therapists (a) learn to naturally and diversely reinforce client target behaviors, (b) hone the capacity to experience intrinsic reinforcement in response to client growth behaviors, (c) practice reinforcing nascent, emerging forms of target behaviors, and (d) courageously decrease CRB1s via differential reinforcement.

Several guidelines help set the stage for offering effective consequation of CRBs. First, it is critical to have conducted a thorough "FAP Rap" (see Chapter 21), ensuring that the client has bought into the FAP rationale for why the therapist will be offering immediate, authentic reinforcement of in-session behaviors. Second, it is helpful to have constructed even a very informal collaborative case conceptualization with a client such that there is explicit agreement between therapist and client regarding the forms and functions of target behaviors. Third, therapists need to themselves possess behaviors that fall within the repertoires of their clients' target behaviors, such that they are well-positioned to identify those behaviors and respond skillfully in their presence. For example, if a client is feeling invalidated by something her therapist said and shuts down, a therapist who is avoidant of conflict is unlikely to discriminate that the client is upset and is engaging in a CRB1 of pulling away and also unlikely to encourage an open discussion of what just happened between them. Thus, without the skills to

DOI: 10.4324/9781032694832-24

address painful feelings in this context, it is less likely that the therapist will be able to unearth and therapeutically address this conflict with the client.

Similarly, if a therapist is disdainful or afraid of client attachment and dependence (e.g., emailing the therapist several times a week, announcing feelings of dread and inability to cope with a therapist's upcoming vacation), the therapist will likely find it difficult to explore the client's feelings in a fruitful way. By contrast, a therapist who is able to practice mindful openness to both their own and the client's reactions in this situation will possess the freedom to explore the client's history of unmet dependency needs, how this learning plays out in current relationships, and the possibility of learning healthier behaviors for expressing attachment and dependency in both the therapeutic relationship and in daily life relationships. Critically, there is no need for or possibility of FAP therapists being unilaterally and deftly skilled in all domains of interpersonal behavior. Rather, of utmost importance is for therapists to be practicing awareness of their own strengths and limitations (including the tender places within their own learning histories that make them prone to seizing up and becoming rigid and ineffective in response to CRBs) and how those interact with their clients' CRBs. With this self-awareness operating, therapists are well-positioned to seek appropriate supervision, training, consultation, and personal therapy as needed (see Chapter 28).

Suppose that, armed with your case conceptualization, you have been practicing Rule 1 and Rule 2, and you spot a CRB2 and want to reinforce it. What should you do? There is an infinite spectrum of potentially reinforcing responses a therapist can offer; ultimately, the essential task is to (a) make an informed guess based on your genuine reaction to the client (in conjunction with what you know of their case conceptualization), (b) observe how they respond (see Rule 4), and then (c) iterate in future attempts. Below, we offer several principles that can serve as a launching pad for considering what kind of reinforcement to offer a client.

Choose natural over arbitrary reinforcement whenever possible

In service of maximizing the reinforcement value of therapist responses and generalizability of CRB2s beyond the therapy relationship into outside life (Rule 5), FAP favors the use of natural versus arbitrary reinforcement (see Chapter 6). If a depressed client emits what you assess to be a CRB2 of enthusiastically describing the book that they have been reading, you could respond with praise: "Way to go! I can tell you're really getting into your behavior activation homework. It's great to see that you're so engaged in treatment." That response may be reinforcing, but for many clients, a more *naturally* reinforcing response could involve responding in a way that is more akin to how the social world typically responds to someone sharing excitement about a book, such as: "This book sounds like a really great read. What did you say the title was? Let me pull out my library list so that I can put it on hold."

Shape successive approximations of target behaviors

When teaching an athlete to pole vault, coaches do not start with the bar at an Olympic height and wait to cheer until the athlete has cleared the bar at that level. To do so would ensure only frustration and discouragement for athletes and coaches alike. Similarly, far from waiting for a fully-formed-treatment-goal-level target behavior to emerge, highly skilled FAP therapists tune into micro-improvements in client behavior and reinforce each iteration of a CRB2 as it develops while also offering evokes (Rule 2) for advancing iterations of it. Suppose in the example above that one of the client's treatment goals is to be able to assert requests more directly. The therapist knows that, later in treatment, it will be a CRB2 for the client to directly say: "I'm really enjoying this book, and I'd like to be able to talk about the themes specifically with you. Would you be interested in reading it?" but that behavior may well be outside of the client's grasp at this time. By spontaneously offering that she will put the book on hold at the library, the therapist is not only delivering reinforcement for today's CRB2 (disclosing authentic emotional reactions associated with values-based behavior), which increases the likelihood that the client may emit a similar or stronger CRB2 in the future, she is also providing a reinforcement sampling opportunity that alerts the client to the possibility that the therapist is interested and willing to share reading material with the client (see below for a further extension of this example). In short, the therapist's task is to identify graded improvements within the client's capability. What is an incremental improvement in terms of the client's current level of functioning? What would be a feasible, but meaningful, stretch for this client?

The necessity of offering reinforcement for incremental improvements raises complications regarding generalizing behavior beyond the therapy room (Rule 5). Specifically, FAP therapists often reinforce CRB2s that may not be reinforced (or may be reinforced differently) by outside others. For example, a very shy client's first attempt at assertiveness may be reinforced by the therapist, even though it was awkward and unlikely to meet with success in the outside world. Likewise, a client's first attempt at spending more time with his wife may be explained away by his wife as "you just want to get me off your back." As such, it can be helpful to discuss both the similarities and differences between the therapy relationship and outside relationships. The therapist may explain that the therapy relationship is an opportunity to practice and improve important interpersonal behaviors before "going on the road" with them. The therapist may also explain that in their role as the client's therapist, they are probably more sensitive to subtle changes and more reinforced by them, because the therapist's only purpose in the relationship is to help the client. It goes without saying that outside relationships are more multidimensional, and relationship partners may require time, patience, and support from the client in their own process of growth before they are able to respond in ways that feel reinforcing to the client. In addition, by being naturally reinforcing of even small improvements over current functioning, the therapist may foster in the client an appreciation for these small changes, such that they become self-reinforcing even in the absence of positive responses from others.

Amplify your own internal reactions

Many of our interpersonal needs coalesce around the receipt of attuned empathy and validation in response to our authentic expressions of self and experience, whether painful, beautiful, or some combination of both. FAP therapists often disclose their own small but significant internal reactions and also mirror those that the client displays. While the essential nature of the reinforcer remains fundamentally unchanged, amplification can help clients discern therapists' private reactions that otherwise may be too subtle to notice. To illustrate, consider the client above who may have difficulty discerning the impact of his affective state on others (a CRB1). His enthusiastic disclosure results in subtle and spontaneous reactions in the therapist that could well be lost without magnification, so the therapist in the example above might go on to say: "As you talk about this book, I can see your eyes sparkling and hear an energy in your voice that's been absent for a long time. It's making me feel excited and actually giving me goosebumps."

Offer clients a window into their positive impact on the therapy relationship and you (as a therapist and a person)

FAP therapists often call on the inherently prosocial nature of the human species in the practice of Rule 3. In general, it feels good to us when we have a positive impact on other humans, and it can be especially powerful for clients (who are, appropriately, typically in the role of receiving aid from their therapists) to know that they have exerted a positive influence on their therapist in some form. With careful attention to client case conceptualization, as well as to maintaining the essential therapeutic frame, a therapist could extend the Rule 3 response above by saying:

> Hearing about what it's been like for you to get back into reading after so many years is making me reflect on hobbies that once brought me joy and that I've allowed to slip into the background over the past decade. I used to really enjoy knitting, and I haven't taken my needles out of the closet in years. You've motivated me to commit to myself and to you that, while you're continuing to read your book this week, I'm going to take out my knitting at least once.

Build a foundation of reinforcement from the outset of therapy—and from the outset of every session

Clients must learn, and re-learn, through experience that the therapist is a reliable source of a variety of forms of reinforcement. Hence, it is critical to offer extensive reinforcement sampling opportunities for clients early on in therapy and observe and talk with clients about how they respond to different forms of reinforcement (i.e., learn their reinforcement repertoires). Though FAP sessions can and will follow many different rhythms, we have often observed that both clients and therapists are able to take larger risks (i.e., emit bigger CRB2s and T2s, respectively) during the latter parts of therapy sessions once both players have become reacquainted with each other as sources of reinforcement. While there is always a risk of skimming the relational surface with chit-chat about the events of a client's week for longer than is wise, some amount of this kind of conversation can serve an important reinforcement sampling function that sets the stage for CRB2s later in the session.

Provide what is requested (when possible)

As noted above, offering attuned empathy and validation is often reinforcing when someone is tacting their lived experience. However, when someone emits a mand (a request), directly or indirectly, the most reinforcing response is typically to fulfill the request if at all possible. It goes without saying that not all client requests are CRB2s and, even when they are, therapists cannot, for all kinds of reasons, grant every client request. Indeed, swimming in the evocative waters of needs that cannot be immediately met in the specifically requested format falls among some of the most challenging and rich therapeutic work we can do. However, in a reasonably simple scenario in which a client for whom making direct requests is a CRB2 requests a feasible scheduling change, a FAP therapist would be apt to agree to the change and highlight the process for added reinforcement:

> I'm really grateful to know that I can count on you to ask me for what you need both because I want to offer it to you whenever I can and because it means I don't have to wonder and worry about what you might be needing since I'm not a mind reader.

Consider inquiring in advance of offering reinforcement that you hope may be powerfully reinforcing

If you are aware, based on the client's case conceptualization, that your intended reinforcement (e.g., evocative autobiographical self-disclosure) may fall flat or, worse, end up punishing the behavior you had hoped to reinforce, it can be prudent to ask for the client's input before proceeding. For example, suppose a client has just engaged in a CRB2 of courageously and skillfully delivering constructive feedback to you about the impact of your T1 of running behind schedule. At the lower end of the risk spectrum, a reinforcing response for many clients might entail offering acknowledgment of your problematic behavior, validation of the client's reaction to it (especially in light of their specific learning history), an apology, and a commitment to work on amending the behavior. Before proceeding with a riskier level of response, a therapist might say:

> Your feedback and the conversation we're having about it is having a really positive impact on me and, if it feels like a good fit to you, I'd like to tell you a little bit more about that impact and why it's so powerful. However, I don't want to divert our attention if your gut says that's not going to feel helpful right now. What feels right to you?

With the client's permission, the therapist might go on to describe how, during the therapist's childhood, feedback was typically delivered in a harsh manner and with little opportunity for growth or connection when a mistake was made. Therefore, the client's skillful delivery of feedback and engagement in a related repairing conversation is having a healing effect on the therapist by helping them grow in ways beyond only becoming more punctual, namely also becoming more self-compassionate and skillfully responsive to receiving constructive feedback. Conversely, if the client were to indicate in response to the therapist's query that they would prefer to maintain a focus on their own experience or to move to a new topic, the therapist would respect that preference—and consider how it may bear on the client's case conceptualization (i.e., however the client responds to the therapist's evoke regarding the availability of therapist self-disclosure, their choice may represent a CRB1, CRB2, or neither).

Responding to CRB1s: the utility of differential reinforcement

Consistent with tenets of behavioral learning, we favor the use of reinforcement and extinction over punishment in shaping client behavior.

Even better, we encourage therapists to use differential reinforcement, a strategy that reinforces CRB2s while diminishing the reinforcement of CRB1s (Cooper et al., 2020). To this end, our first line of defense against CRB1s is typically to identify the function of the CRB1 collaboratively with the client such that when the CRB1 emerges, the therapist can focus on blocking the (often negative) reinforcement that is typically available and evoking an associated CRB2 (which will be positively reinforced upon its occurrence).

If reassurance seeking is a CRB1 for a client who, while looking at the floor, says to their therapist: "You must think I'm a terrible person for having an affair," their therapist might respond:

> I can see how deeply this shame is cutting into you, and it's piercing places in my own heart that remind me of decisions of all kinds I've made that I'm not proud of. Would you be willing to meet my eyes for a moment and hold these painful parts of our common humanity together?

Continuing the example of the depressed client for whom talking enthusiastically about a book was initially a CRB2, several weeks or months later, the client's expression of enthusiasm about a book might no longer represent a CRB2 and, indeed, might actually represent an indirectly expressed wish for the therapist to join them in reading the book. At this future time, the therapist might have the following interaction in response to the client's enthusiastic discussion of the book he is reading (now a CRB1):

> *T:* As you're talking about these meaningful themes from your life that are showing up in this novel, I have this feeling that maybe there's an unspoken question sitting right at the tip of your tongue. Is there something you'd like to ask me?" (Rule 3 [Extinction] + Rule 2: the therapist compassionately withholds the reinforcement that may be maintaining the problematic behavior and instead offers an evoke for a CRB2.)
> *C:* Well, I would really like to know your thoughts about the book because I've really been enjoying it."[CRB2].

> *T:* It's so helpful to hear you say directly that you'd like to talk about my reactions to the book. I feel like you're really inviting me to participate, and it makes me eager to have those conversations with you. While it may take a little time, I can commit to reading at least a couple of chapters and sharing my thoughts with you. (Rule 3 [Reinforcing the alternative behavior, a CRB2].)

Although FAP therapists favor extinction, there is an essential place for therapist responses that are more immediately aimed at reducing the strength and/or frequency of problematic behaviors (i.e., in behavioral terms, the punishment of CRB1s). Addressing CRB1s often involves making therapeutic use of negative personal reactions representative of the client's community, such as, "It's hard for me to track what's really important to you when you go on long tangents." Common CRB1s to which therapists may respond with directly punishing responses include those that have an important negative impact on the therapist to the extent that it harms the therapy relationship (or otherwise impedes the therapist's ability to provide the client with effective care) and those to which the therapist has an aversive response that likely reflects what people in the client's outside life are experiencing. Of note, therapists must possess sufficient self-awareness to be reasonably certain that in any particular situation they are a relevant model of others in the client's life (and seek consultation when uncertain) versus their response reflecting only an outgrowth of their own learning history (personal and/or cultural) that would be unlikely to be relevant within the client's local social world. It is also critical to underscore that therapists must consequate CRB1s in the context of: (a) their evident caring and concern for the client; (b) their belief in the client's ability to produce more adaptive behavior; (c) a conceptualization of the client's problems that relies on an understanding of relevant historical and environmental factors rather than on something being inherently wrong inside the client; and (d) the client's concurrence that CRB1s are in-session problems connected with daily life problems.

It is optimal to address CRB1s after a strong therapeutic relationship has formed, the client has experienced a great deal of natural positive reinforcement from the therapist, and the client has given permission for the therapist to do so. For example, a therapist might inquire in advance with a client: "We've talked about how it's a problem for people to track you when you go off on tangents. Is it okay for me to interrupt you when you do that with me?" If possible, it is best to address or block a CRB1 after the client has already has emitted a CRB2 counterpart at some point. For example, a therapist can say, "You know how sometimes you are really able to let yourself feel and express your sadness with me? What's stopping you from doing that right now?" Remember that your tone of voice and other non-verbal cues (leaning forward, moving your chair closer) can also act as reinforcers. In general, we call for compassionate responses to CRB1s unless that has not worked in the past or the CRB1 calls for a sterner tone.

The therapist, when responding to CRB1s, is in fact not so much trying to punish CRB1s as they are trying to evoke CRB2s, and if the therapist determines that it is unlikely that the client will successfully emit CRB2s in the session, it is probably a good idea to back away from FAP moves altogether rather than increasing the aversive qualities of the session by continuing to punish the client's behavior. Therapists must not forget that a side effect of using punishment is that aversive properties of the procedures are often transferred to those who administered it. Clients in fact may be likely to drop out of therapy if sessions are dominated by responding to CRB1s rather than CRB2s. Only in rare cases, for example when the client's behavior is life-threatening, should a therapist persist in punishing CRB1s in the absence of CRB2s. Based on all the precautions mentioned above, our foremost recommendation is to use differential reinforcement whenever possible. As such, when responding to CRB1s with extinction or punishment procedures, it is essential to be concurrently evoking CRB2s and reinforcing any and all forms of improved behavior.

In sum, the strategic application of authentic reinforcement is the preeminent Rule 3 procedure. Indeed, evidence from multiple studies suggests that the reinforcement of CRB2s is a primary mechanism of therapeutic change in FAP (see Kanter et al., 2017 for review). A simple rule of thumb for the FAP therapist: When in doubt, offer reinforcement—and observe what happens next (Rule 4).

Noticing our effect (Rule 4)

To attempt the strategic reinforcement that characterizes Rule 3 without consistently practicing awareness of the actual outcomes of these attempts would be akin to rowing a boat while looking only at the rudder, never looking up at the horizon to assess the impact of your steering efforts. Rule 4 reminds us to observe the actual impact of our endeavors to shape client behavior so that we do not inadvertently end up reinforcing problematic behaviors and punishing or extinguishing growth behaviors—at least not over extended periods of time!

The practice of Rule 4 ideally takes place both implicitly (via silent therapist observations of client behavior following Rule 3 moves) and explicitly (via collaborative exchanges of feedback with the client). In addition, it is conducted on both the macro level (i.e., are the strength and/or frequency of CRB2s increasing across weeks and months of treatment?) and micro level (i.e., what is the immediate impact of the therapist's Rule 3 response on client behavior right now in the session?). Suppose a client who typically struggles to acknowledge when they have made a mistake (CRB1) emits a CRB2 of apologizing for having been brusque with the therapist during the previous session. In an attempt to offer reinforcement, a FAP therapist might be inclined to respond along the lines of: "Thank you so much for acknowledging that your tone was a bit harsh last week. I did feel hurt that you were pushing me away, and it means a lot to me that our relationship matters enough to you that you'd want to apologize and repair it with me. I'm excited that I can feel the trust building in our relationship." For some clients at some moments in therapy, this response might feel highly reinforcing of the emotional risk they had taken to apologize, and they might continue emitting CRB2s (e.g., expressing appreciation for the therapist's gracious response, mirroring the feeling of burgeoning emotional safety in the therapy relationship, or sharing previously undisclosed learning history related to their struggles in the process of rupture and repair). By contrast, other clients, depending on learning history as well as the current stage of therapy, might experience the therapist's acknowledgment of having felt hurt as threatening or overwhelming and begin emitting CRB1s in response (e.g., shutting down and saying very little, lashing out with sarcasm, or avoiding by changing the topic). Either way, by looking up at the horizon and becoming curious about *what happens next* after offering a contingency, a FAP therapist is well-equipped to adjust the rudder of the boat so as not to go too far off course.

Therapists may gather some information by observing the client's verbal and non-verbal behavior following a Rule 3 move. In addition, it is important to inquire directly at times with the client about their experience of your Rule 3 interventions, both in specific moments and in general: "What was it like when I told you how moved I was by what you'd just said?" "How is it for you when I tear up in response to something you share?" "What does it feel like when I say I'm proud of you?" "I'm feeling really excited and expressing a lot of enthusiasm right now, and I'm not sure how it's landing with you." Of note, this explicit engagement of Rule 4 is also an evoke (Rule 2): The therapist is asking the client to offer feedback (FIAT Class B), and, regardless of the specific content of the feedback that the client delivers, the therapist should also be interested in the possibility that the client's response may comprise CRB1s or CRB2s (or both). Using a bridging questionnaire routinely between sessions is an excellent way to ensure that clients are consistently provided an opportunity to offer feedback (as well as other essential information) about the impact of the previous session and the therapy process in general.

The reality is that we will inevitably fail sometimes in our strategic application of contingencies, in the form of both unconscious errors and conscious but ill-fated Rule 3 attempts. Yet, so long as we engage Rule 4 on both micro- and macro-levels, each instance of deviation from the charted course offers valuable opportunities, including understanding the client and their case conceptualization more thoroughly and strengthening the therapeutic alliance. With a consistent Rule 4 practice, we can ensure that the therapy boat never gets too far off track before a course correction, ripe with therapeutic possibilities itself, can be applied.

24

Generalizing and discriminating (Rule 5)

"I'd love others to be like you outside!" This statement is commonly heard from clients who have experienced the empowering effects of a reinforcing therapeutic relationship in FAP. Encouraging clients to display CRB2s in contexts other than therapy is achievable through the promotion of generalization and discrimination processes. From a behavioral perspective, generalization and discrimination are part of a continuum. Generalization is defined as "the occurrence of relevant behavior under different, non-training conditions (i.e., across subjects, settings, people, behaviors, and/or time) without the scheduling of the same events in those conditions as were scheduled in the training conditions" (Stokes & Baer, 1977, p. 350). Discrimination refers to the process by which a behavior is elicited in response to one stimulus but not to another (McIlvane, 2013).

In FAP, therapists use Rule 5 to help clients transfer their progress from sessions to daily life (generalization) and to identify the contexts in which their progress is more likely to be reinforced or punished (discrimination). To achieve this, therapists encourage clients to develop functional verbal descriptions of the contextual cues and reinforcers that control their behaviors (CRB3). Learning to distinguish between different types of social environments may be the most effective tool for sustaining progress and reducing relapses. Two strategies are particularly useful for promoting generalization and discrimination: (a) drawing parallels between behaviors in sessions and in daily life, and (b) aiding clients to formulate tracking rules that describe the contingencies controlling interpersonal behaviors.

Parallels between in-session and daily life behaviors

Out-to-in parallels take place when daily-life events are related to corresponding in-session situations, and in-to-out parallels occur when in-session events are related to corresponding daily-life events. These parallels may facilitate the generalization of gains (Rule 5) made in the

DOI: 10.4324/9781032694832-26

client-therapist relationship to daily life as well as assist in identifying CRB (Rule 1). Both types of parallels are important, and a good FAP session may involve considerable weaving between daily-life and in-session content through multiple in-to-out and out-to-in parallels.

Facilitating generalization is essential in FAP. Below is an example based on an interaction between a FAP therapist and her client "Alicia" who participated in a 20-session treatment for depression and smoking cessation. They are talking about an out-to-in parallel that Alicia is struggling with regarding her pulling away once she knows someone cares about her.

T: You know how I've said to you a number of times in our work together that our relationship is very, very important, and that it's a microcosm of your outside life relationships. [Rule 2. The therapist has been hypothesizing that Alicia canceling her recent sessions due to back pain may be a CRB1 involving avoidance of the closeness that has been increasing in their therapeutic relationship.]

C: Yeah, I was thinking about that, and I kind of wrote about it on my session bridging sheet. When I think back to the relation-ships I've been in, all my boyfriends, I really relish the pursuit, but once they turn around and start liking me, I go "Yuck." Then I feel smothered. I realized I did that in this relationship too in a way [CRB3.]

T: With me? [Rule 1.]

C: Yeah, it was like the excitement in the beginning, everything's new, then you really focused on me and turned your attention to me, and I froze. And I don't know why at a point when people reciprocate the energy, I'm putting into it, then I freak out [CRB3.]

T: Close relationships involving intimacy can bring about a lot of hurt, which you've certainly experienced in your relationships with men. So, it makes sense that you might want to be cautious and pull away. That gives you more of a sense of control over the relationship, but it can also bring about the very outcome that you are trying to avoid [a Rule 5 interpretation]. It's so important that you can say this out loud, it's incredible, because I certainly felt you freaking out [Rule 3, natural reinforcement of what she is saying].

C: When relationships get to the stage where they matter to me, I have some kind of psychic time gauge, I have to reject it before I get rejected. If I sit it out and I'm convinced I won't be rejected right off the bat, I'm able to recommit myself [CRB3.]

T: This is really important. I can't wait for you to get into a relationship, have this issue come up, and talk about it. I can't emphasize enough how connecting it is to have someone tell you what's going on, to have you tell me, this whole conversation we are having is just awesome [Rule 3, more natural reinforcement; Rule 5, encouraging an in-to-out parallel.]

Providing functional analytically informed interpretations can help clients in two ways. First, the functional interpretations can lead to a prescription, instruction, or rule. The interpretation, "You are acting toward your wife like you did toward your mother," can easily be taken as a prescription: "Treat your wife more fairly since she obviously is not your mother, and your relationship will improve" Second, it can enhance the salience of controlling variables and increase reinforcement density by acting as a "signal." For example, a female client learns that the reason she feels rejected at times during the session is a function of the therapist's attentiveness level and that this attentiveness is related to how late in the day it is. As a result, the client is in better contact (she notices that the therapist is less attentive when she sees him late in the day) and then experiences less aversiveness when he is inattentive.

The verbal repertoire to be developed by therapists involves statements that relate events during the session to the relationship symbolized by Sd R → Sr. This represents operant behavior in which (1) Sd is the discriminative stimulus or prior situation whose influence over the occurrence of R varies with the reinforcement history; (2) R is the response or operant behavior, which is influenced by the Sd; and (3) Sr is the reinforcement or effect of the response on the environment. For example,

When I asked you how you are feeling about our therapeutic relationship (Sd), you responded by talking about your therapy goals (R), which is another topic that you know I'm interested in. I rewarded your avoidance by talking about therapy goals (Sr).

As a general strategy, it is useful to interpret client statements in terms of functional relationships, learning history, and behavior. Downplaying mentalistic and nonbehavioral entities, such as inadequate motivation, low self-esteem, lack of ego strength, and fear of success, and instead emphasizing behavioral interpretations and history are useful to clients because attention is directed to external factors that lend themselves to therapeutic interventions.

Formulation of tracking rules

FAP interventions focus on continuously providing contingent rein-forcement to decrease CRB1s and promote CRB2s. This exchange occurs in the presence of specific Sd introduced by the therapist during sessions. These contextual cues may be topographically or functionally equivalent to those encountered in the clients' daily lives. However, there are times when Sd for CRB2s rarely or never occur outside of therapy sessions. In such situations, the likelihood of clients receiv-ing reinforcement for exhibiting CRB2s outside of therapy is low. To enhance the likelihood of identifying contexts where clients' improve-ments are effectively acknowledged, therapists might facilitate in-ses-sion tracking. *Tracking* is "rule-governed behavior under the control of the apparent correspondence between the rule and the arrangement of the world" (Törneke et al., 2008, p. 148). Specifically, in-session tracking is recommended to encourage clients to functionally describe factors within the session that facilitate and strengthen their CRB2s. Through such tracking (also known as a type of CRB3s), clients can learn to identify out-of-session factors that share functions with thera-peutic contextual cues and thus support their progress.

In Alicia's case, the therapist can support her in identifying Sd and Sr in their therapeutic relationship that facilitate intimate interactions.

> *T:* Today, I've felt a real connection with you. I see all the effort you've put into being honest with me. It must have been chal-lenging for you to keep the conversation going instead of jok-ing or changing the subject.
> *C:* Well, you didn't make it easy. I actually found myself wanting to change the topic, but you kept me focused.

T: What did I do that encouraged you to share what was in your heart? [Rule 2.]

C: You were so kind and gentle; I just couldn't hide from you. You asked me the right questions about my fears, my avoidance, my old patterns. Somehow, you managed the perfect balance between challenge and care [CRB3.]

T: Oh, that means a lot to me. Providing both care and challenge, engaging in extraordinary relationships, is exactly what I'm looking for. Could you pinpoint anything specific I did? [Rule 2.]

C: You asked how I felt, listened attentively, showed genuine care, and respected my opinions. And you didn't let me dodge the issues; you stayed with me through them [CRB3.]

T: And when you shared those vulnerable parts of yourself with me, what did I do?

C: You were there for me, with no judgment, no advice, just taking care of me [CRB3.]

T: Can you then describe to me the formula for intimacy? [Rule 2.]

C: Well, I guess it is sharing what I'm most afraid of with someone who really pays attention to me and who cares for me... or something of that sort [CRB3.]

T: I think that is a great description of what just happened between us. Can we look for these other people outside who offer that to you? [Rule 5.]

In the dialogue above, the therapist asked various questions to aid Alicia in identifying what therapist's behaviors facilitate her display of vulnerable behaviors in session. The therapist's goal is to assist Alicia in independently formulating functional verbal rules or tracks. Encouraging clients to track the contingencies can facilitate the discrimination of factors that naturally control their behavior. Adopting this strategy promotes the development of flexible behavioral repertoires over rigid, therapist-prescribed rules (Pliance). This flexibility proves beneficial for adjusting strategies that may not be effective and for maintaining progress in the absence of the therapist.

25

A logical therapeutic interaction in FAP

FAP's five rules may be applied flexibly and functionally, thus application of FAP may look quite different from one client to another, because each client's CRBs and what is reinforcing those CRBs may be quite different. In our experience, however, we have found that some powerful FAP interactions follow a logical in-session sequence. Here we describe some commonalities that appear across the authors' experiences of these powerful in-session FAP sequences. An important aspect of this 12-step sequence is that FAP's five rules are instantiated in order from Rule 1 to Rule 5 as the interaction proceeds. Thus, the interaction is a demonstration of FAP in total. Specifying the interaction at the level of the moment-to-moment therapist-client interaction may be helpful for both training and research purposes (Tsai et al., 2014).

The interaction assumes that a good, strong FAP relationship is already in place. The therapist: a) is deeply in touch with the contingencies of reinforcement that have shaped his or her client, b) is feeling deep compassion for the client's history of wounds and losses, and c) is aware of the client's CRB1s and CRB2s in the context of this history (Rule 1). In session, the therapist is also maintaining strong connection with the client using eye contact and body language that conveys compassion. Finally, in addition to contingently reinforcing improvements, the therapist is providing a solid and explicit foundation of validation for what the client is disclosing both in the moment and over the course of therapy.

In this context, here now is the logical interaction. It starts with the client and therapist discussing daily life material.

1. **Therapist out-to-in parallel.** The therapist provides an out-to-in parallel (Rule 1), drawing a parallel between events in the client's daily life and what is happening in the therapy relationship: "The

DOI: 10.4324/9781032694832-27

way you are talking about protecting yourself with your husband, do you feel that you have to protect yourself with me, too?"

2. **Client confirmation of the accuracy of the parallel.** The client confirms the accuracy of the parallel: "Yes." Of course, sometimes parallels will not be accurate, and that is fine. Not everything in the client's life needs to have an in-session parallel in FAP.

3. **Therapist evokes CRB.** With the parallel confirmed, the therapist evokes CRB (Rule 2) with respect to the behavior: "How about right now, could you drop your guard and be a little more real with me? I'd really like to see it."

4. **Client emits CRB1.** Typically, the first time CRB is evoked, it will be CRB1 of avoidance: "I don't know, that would be really hard." Of course, ideally there will be few CRB1s and more CRB2s instead. Although the therapist is never hoping for CRB1, s/he is prepared for them.

5. **Therapist contingently responds to CRB1.** In response, the therapist contingently responds to the CRB1 (Rule 3), by blocking the avoidance and re-presenting the evocative question: "I understand how hard it is for you. Still, I think you are strong, and I believe you can let your guard down a bit right now. How about if you take a breath and try?"

   Loops in which steps 4 and 5 are repeated several times are common in the logical FAP interaction. The client avoids, the therapist blocks it and tries again to evoke CRB2; the client continues to avoid, and the therapist continues compassionately to gently block and evoke. Essentially, an "extinction struggle" is occurring: Will the client's CRB1 avoidance behavior extinguish or will the therapist's attempts to block CRB1 and evoke CRB2 extinguish? The therapist should be gauging the client's tolerance for this extended struggle, because it is important in FAP for the session to stay positive and constructive, to focus on CRB2s, not CRB1s, and thus to view even very small improvements in the client's behavior as CRB2s.

6. **Client emits CRB2.** The client engages in CRB2: "Well, I appreciate you saying that. I do want to be more genuine here; it is just so hard for me to be real" (crying). When CRB2 such as this takes place, the fundamental moment in FAP has occurred.

7. **Therapist contingently responds to CRB2.** The therapist contingently responds to the CRB2 with natural reinforcement (Rule 3):

   Well, I really feel you right now, my heart is completely open to you, and I am filled with compassion for what you are going through. When you cry like this, I have this exquisite sense of your pain and all you have gone through. While I know you don't like to cry in front of people, right now you are doing so makes me feel closer to you, and I will not hurt you.

   Much of FAP training is about helping FAP therapists respond well to CRB2s—genuinely, compassionately, fully, and immediately. Each FAP therapist will have his or her own style in doing so, and the response above should not be emulated as the "correct" response. We do believe; however, it is important to notice that the response above is full and long. We want the reinforcing response to be extremely salient, clear, and unambiguous to the client. We want the client to have no doubt how the therapist feels in response to the CRB2.

8. **Client engages in more CRB2.** The client emits more CRB2: "When you say that it is really hard to hear, but somehow, I believe you (crying more)." When clients respond to the therapist's attempt to do Rule 3 with more CRB2, that is confirmation that Rule 3 was effective (Rule 4). The best interactions in FAP are when loops occur in which steps 7 and 8 repeat: the therapist reinforces CRB2, the client engages in more CRB2, the therapist reinforces the new CRB2, and the client continues to engage in more CRB2. In this way, CRB2s quickly and powerfully can be shaped and strengthened. Oftentimes, these interactions are characterized by both client and therapist vulnerability, in which both are feeling the discomfort that comes with true rapid increases in intimacy.

9. **Therapist engages in Rule 4.** The therapist asks about the effect of his or her response to the client (Rule 4): "So how was all that for you?" The therapist should not rush into this step; in fact, it could happen during the next session. The primary issue is that the Step 7–8 loop in which CRB2s are shaped should come to a natural end and not be rushed. Once the interaction has naturally stopped, the remaining steps in the interaction are about "processing" and generalizing the interaction.

10. **Client indicates that the interaction was reinforcing.** The client suggests that the therapist was reinforcing: "I feel relieved, good." This processing of the interaction is helpful in assessing what is reinforcing to the client, but the therapist should keep in mind that in FAP, reinforcement is defined functionally as that which increases client behavior, not by what the client reports s/he likes. Therefore, Rule 4 primarily is about observing the impact of the therapist's response on the client's behavior over time. Nonetheless, immediate feedback on the impact of the interaction, as per this step, is often useful to the therapist.

11. **Therapist engages in Rule 5.** The therapist provides a functional description of the interaction, an in-to-out parallel, and homework assignment based on the interaction (Rule 5):

    Well, it seems to me that what just happened is that you took a risk and let your guard down. I responded by letting you know how I felt when I saw you do that, which in turn helped you open up even more, and now you feel relieved and good [functional interpretation]. I am wondering what would happen if you were like this more often with your spouse [in-to-out parallel]? Do you think we can spend a few minutes now talking about what you can do differently with your spouse [leading to homework assignment]?

12. **Client expresses willingness to engage in homework.** The final step in the interaction is the client expressing willingness to try the new behavior in his or her daily life.

Overall, this logical interaction consists of three phases. First, with steps 1, 2, and 3, the issue is awareness of CRBs and bringing CRBs into the room. Then, with steps 48, the issue is shaping CRB2s—this is the heart of FAP. Finally, the third phase consists of processing and generalizing the interaction. When all 12 steps occur, we expect FAP interactions to be more powerful and lasting than when the interaction is only partially completed. Exploring this hypothesis is an important research direction for FAP.

26

Loss of connection: Working with grief in FAP

Loss is a part of the human experience, loss due to death, divorce, moving, estrangement, or any instance of disconnection after connection results in an alteration of what is usual for a person. A client can be heartbroken, shut down, barely able to face the world, and/or can also be relieved, and even joyful, focused on treasuring life. And everything in between. The use of functional analysis in understanding and helping with grief offers an openness to human experience that can aid in responding sensitively and meaningfully to a client no matter where they are in their grief, and no matter what their loss means to them. Similarly, the FAP therapist who is in contact with their own losses is also changed and has been altered (more open, more closed, and everything in between) when doing clinical work with suffering or even joyful people. And post loss, humans have unique ways of responding to the loss: some feeling profoundly alone; some perhaps feeling a spiritual and actual connection to the person who has died; and/or an opening to common humanity. The beauty of FAP is that any and all experiences may be explored in the therapeutic relationship. It is also a real, in-vivo experience of grief being a bridge, a path to closeness, not a brick wall between people as one who is bereaved may feel.

The therapy relationship in all therapies has a beginning, a middle, and an end. Sometimes these phases are clear and identified, sometimes endings and changes are unplanned and unexpected. In FAP, one thing is clear, which is that a relationship begins with two strangers, and over time, a relationship is developed that we hope becomes deeply meaningful to both client and therapist. This experience, a "laboratory of love," is an in-vivo experience of the meaning and connection that can grow when sharing grief with another person. Clients who might conclude that they can never love again, can learn, in therapy, that unbeknownst to them, their heart is not done loving and opening

DOI: 10.4324/9781032694832-28

and creating connections with another. And in FAP, one can explore that taking risks and growing close to one's therapist involves the same kinds of intimacy repertoires that are needed in one's daily life.

Saying goodbye in therapy can also be a deeply evocative time to explore past goodbyes and losses. How have losses been navigated in the past, what is the client proud of, what kinds of regrets may be there? How can the goodbye in therapy grow skills for future goodbyes? How can the therapist and client talk about what happens post-therapy, how memories, longing, and absence can be felt and held compassionately?

27

Termination

The end of relationships often incites powerful and mixed emotions both in and outside of therapy. We have all experienced relational endings, small and large, that were incompletely acknowledged and/or emotionally jagged, whether casually skipped over in a morass of covert avoidance (e.g., "We'll see each other again—I'll call you soon!"), vehemently pushed away in the silence and/or anger of conflict, or traumatically omitted by sudden loss. Ideally, treatment termination provides a forum for a corrective emotional experience wherein the emotional complexity of saying goodbye, including all the relevant history it elicits for the client, can be conjointly named and held with reverence.

Because we wish to upend the tendency to avoid endings, it is wise to, somewhat ironically, acknowledge the inevitable ending of therapy right from the very beginning and set the expectation with clients that saying goodbye is an active and essential element of the treatment that the therapist is offering. Some FAP therapists even describe the importance of having an intentional termination process in their disclosure statements and highlight this topic during the intake process. Just as there is no standard treatment duration in FAP, there is no set number of sessions needed to process termination; timing should vary depending on the duration of treatment and client case conceptualization. In time-limited therapy, the client and therapist may know at the outset that treatment will consist of only 20 sessions or a given number of months. In long-term treatment, termination may be expected to occur once the client and therapist agree that goals have been met or that sufficient progress has been made. Regardless, the topic should be raised well in advance of probable termination so that both participants can have a contextually appropriate number of sessions to discuss the ending of therapy (see Tsai et al., 2017 for a detailed description of the rationale, supporting evidence, and procedures associated with FAP terminations).

In brief, termination presents an opportunity for clients (and therapists) to expand their behavioral repertoires related to saying goodbye. Therapists carry their own histories associated with relational endings, so it is essential that they practice awareness of how this learning has shaped their own behaviors in the setting of saying goodbye to be able to, with awareness of the client's case conceptualization, shepherd the therapy relationship through a "good goodbye." Therapists may initiate a conversation about termination by saying something such as: "Endings and loss are a part of life and relationships, and the therapeutic relationship allows for a unique opportunity to end an important relationship thoughtfully by acknowledging the impact we've had on each other." One question to explore in detail is: "For many clients, the end of therapy brings up feelings and memories of previous transitions and losses. What thoughts and feelings do endings in general bring up for you? What thoughts and feelings are you having about the ending of our therapy relationship?" Ideally, the therapist will have been constructing a flexible and iterative case conceptualization of the client throughout the course of treatment, such that they are able to determine if the client's responses to these prompts (Rule 2) are CRB1s or CRB2s, respond contingently (Rule 3), and continue evoking accordingly (Rule 2). However, humans are complex, and case conceptualization is a necessarily evolving and often murky process, so termination may well elicit and evoke behavior that does not fit neatly into the therapist's exisiting understanding of the client's CRB1s and CRB2s. When such surprises emerge, there is fruitful opportunity for interactions with the client that lead to an even deeper understanding of the client, their learning history, and the meaning of the therapy relationship, including and beyond the goodbye to it.

A FAP therapist may invite clients to exchange end-of-therapy letters with them. Both the writing and reciprocal sharing of such letters can be an important component of the treatment consolidation and parting process. Both letters may include a description of progress made, what the therapist and client appreciate about each other, reminiscences of interactions that were especially moving during therapy, and what the therapist and client will remember or take away from the therapy. The therapist may also choose to highlight in their letter to the client what growth they hope the client will maintain and continue, their wishes for the client, and parting advice. Clients should have a clear sense of the ways in which they are special and clarity about the gifts they have to contribute to their relationships, their communities, and perhaps the world. Providing clients with a closing letter gives them something tangible to take away from therapy and a concrete reminder of their progress and of the therapeutic relationship. Even if the therapist and client do not choose to exchange written letters, these prompts are all important fodder for conversation throughout the termination process.

The final chapter of FAP is a time to consolidate gains and to ensure that the new, adaptive behaviors that have germinated within the therapeutic relationship have taken root in the client's outside life (Rule 5), while also setting the stage for this growth to continue (i.e., relapse prevention). Fundamentally, it is a chance for the client to practice the very same courageous behaviors that the therapy has targeted within the highly evocative context of losing an important relationship. This collaborative embrace of saying a meaningful goodbye creates a model of how it is possible to approach the ending of a relationship with love and openness to the rich, multidimensional emotional orbit that is inevitable when we allow ourselves to confront the finitude of life and the relationships that we inhabit within it.

Supervision and training

As experiential as it is didactic, FAP supervision and training emphasize the learning of clinical knowledge and skills as well as the self-development of the therapist that is required to competently implement these tools in the therapy room. There are ten core competencies relevant to conducting FAP that guide training regardless of the specific level and setting:

1. Creating a behavior analytic case conceptualization
2. Understanding CRBs as functional classes, not topographically specific forms of behavior
3. Identifying CRBs (Rule 1)
4. Responding to CRB1s effectively (Rule 3)
5. Evoking CRBs (Rule 2)
6. Responding to CRB2s effectively (Rule 3)
7. Expressing a naturally reinforcing repertoire of warmth, trust-establishment, risk-taking, and self-disclosure
8. Demonstrating awareness of reinforcement impact (Rule 4)
9. Demonstrating awareness of T1s and T2s
10. Providing functional analytically informed interpretations and implementing generalization strategies (Rule 5)

Together, these competencies delineate a conceptual framework for understanding the FAP supervision and training process (Callaghan, 2006b; Kohlenberg & Tsai, 1991; Tsai et al., 2009; Follette & Callaghan, 1995).

Consistent with supervision across all theoretical orientations, the first goal of FAP supervision and training is to increase the supervisee's knowledge base and critical and conceptual clinical thinking skills. This goal is accomplished via modeling of competence, specific instructions

DOI: 10.4324/9781032694832-30

(including reading assignments), goal setting, and feedback on performance (Milne & James, 2000). The FAP knowledge base consists of a verbal repertoire for describing the important features of the therapeutic process. For example, supervisees learn to: (a) develop a case conceptualization in order to understand which client behaviors may be CRB1s and CRB2s (Rule 1); (b) evoke (Rule 2) and naturally reinforce CRB2s (Rule 3); and (c) conduct a functional analysis of T1s and T2s that occur during treatment and supervision.

The second goal of FAP supervision and training is to directly shape and increase the effectiveness of therapist behaviors related to noticing, evoking, and strengthening CRB2s. These therapist behaviors are contingency-shaped and, unlike improvements in the FAP knowledge base, improvements in contingency-shaped behavior can occur outside of awareness. This sort of knowledge is described in everyday language as "deep," "emotional," and "intuitive" (Skinner, 1974).

In FAP supervision, therapist behavior is learned through direct exposure to an intense interpersonal relationship with the supervisor, in which emitting and noticing important behaviors (T1s and T2s) occur. Safran and Muran (2001) similarly suggest that in supervision, as in therapy, all interactions take place within a relational context. They contend that supervision should include in-vivo experiential opportunities because learning primarily at a conceptual level is insufficient. The contrast between intellectual knowing versus emotional knowing through supervision is aptly described by one supervisee:

> Many other supervisors tried to teach me to be emotionally present with my clients. But I am finding that going there is something I do heart-first. To do this task, I needed more than hearing it in supervision, reading it in an article, or watching it on a video. I needed to experience it myself, in-vivo, within the supervisory relationship. That, for me, is the core of FAP and FAP supervision that is transforming me and my work.

The supervision methods described below delineate a range of ways supervisors can create powerful relationships with their supervisees. Such relationships aim to create profound moments in which supervisees experience large personal gains that make them more effective FAP therapists.

Create a "sacred" space for supervision

Just as FAP therapists create a sacred therapeutic space for their clients, FAP supervisors create a similar sacred space for their supervisees. As stated in Chapter 16, a "sacred" space is exclusively dedicated to some person or special purpose, protected by sanction from incursion. Whether or not it is labeled in this way, the key is that FAP supervisors create an environment in which supervisees can feel safe and deeply cared for as they learn how to implement FAP. Just as in therapy, this mission is achieved by establishing a genuine relationship, explicitly describing the rationale for supervision, and maximizing positive reinforcement during supervision. Functionally, the more sacred and positively reinforcing the supervisory space, the more likely the supervisee will take risks, leading to transformational changes in repertoires.

Focus on in-vivo work when appropriate

It is important in FAP supervision to focus on in-vivo work that is relevant to the supervisee's growth as a therapist. This is done through contingent natural reinforcement of supervisee target behaviors in the context of the sacred space and the real relationship between the supervisor and the supervisee. The supervisor may evoke and naturally reinforce key supervisee target behaviors that apply to FAP, such as being aware, being courageous, and being therapeutically loving. FAP supervisors and supervisees should together determine what the supervisees' T1s and T2s are, and the supervisor should be sensitive to these as they occur in the supervisory relationship. Because the frame of supervision is more flexible than the frame of therapy, supervisors may choose to disclose in more detail than they typically would with a client information about their own T1s and T2s (as well as S1s and S2s in the context of supervision) with the supervisee and may be quicker to invite supervisees to be explicitly reinforcing of the supervisor's improvements as well. Typical T2 targets in supervision include decreasing avoidance and increasing courage. Decreased avoidance by therapists involves taking judicious risks; facing one's own fear and asking others to do the same; regulated experiencing and expression of feelings (such as caring, sadness, anger; FIAT Class E), building emotionally intimate connections (FIAT D); asking someone who is in pain to do difficult things, such as respecting limits (FIAT Class A); giving and receiving uncomfortable feedback (FIAT Class B), and welcoming conflict or disagreement (FIAT C).

By responding to supervisees' T1s and T2s, the FAP supervisor also provides a model to the supervisee of the process of implementing FAP rules (being aware of CRBs, evoking CRBs, naturally reinforcing CRB2s, being aware of one's impact, and providing functional analytic interpretations that support the generalization of improved behavior). For example, being therapeutically loving is an important aspect of Rule 3, equated with being naturally reinforcing and with being reinforced by your supervisees' improvements and successes. Being therapeutically loving is a broad class of therapy behaviors that supervisors can model contextually, and such training is likely to be relevant to supervisees' therapeutic work. The supervisory relationship can become emotionally intimate and profound as supervisors demonstrate therapeutic love. Ideally, supervisees' experience of this process facilitates their engagement in a parallel, contextually appropriate version of it with clients.

Thus, FAP supervisors are authentic in describing their thoughts and feelings to their supervisees. They see, evoke, value, and reinforce their supervisees' best qualities, which may evoke feedback from supervisees such as: "You mirror back to me the best of who I am, and you see the best of who I am capable of becoming." Like FAP therapy, the intensity of FAP supervision will vary depending on the needs and repertoires of the supervisees and may evolve over time as supervisees grow and eventually graduate from supervision (see Chapter 14 for ethics and precautions).

FAP compassion fatigue

Because providing FAP requires consistent, ongoing, exquisitely sensitive attunement to clients' emotional experiences and consistent emotional risk-taking on the part of both therapists and clients, FAP therapists may be at an especially high risk of experiencing compassion fatigue (see Sinclair et al., 2017 for a review of this phenomenon in healthcare providers) in the absence of sufficient self-care and supportive surrounding social support. Even if following a somewhat protocol-driven FAP approach, there is no way to provide competent FAP without bringing forward (in a contextually appropriate form guided by the client's case conceptualization) the authentic and vulnerable self of the therapist. The topographies of therapist vulnerability will vary widely across therapists, clients, and phases of treatment and must also be responsive to the availability of a therapist's emotional, physical, mental, and spiritual resources during any given session. Yet, within all this flexibility, the essential core of FAP requires therapists to engage in an ongoing practice of emotional awareness, attunement, and risk-taking that necessitates an ongoing restoration of emotional reserves in the therapist.

While the particular strategies that satisfy needs for such restoration are as ideographic as CRBs, seasoned FAP therapists often report that participation in the following activities may be helpful in various doses at different times over the course of a career: peer consultation with trusted colleagues (whether one-on-one or in a team), nourishing interpersonal relationships in outside life, physical activity, spiritual practices, personal therapy, and prioritizing time for rest and play (on a daily and weekly basis, and also in the form of taking vacations from clinical work). In the professional realm, it may be helpful at times to diversify the populations with whom the therapist works, diversify other professional activities (e.g., lead a training, try writing a book, start supervising a student—or conversely take a break from any of these activities), and seek additional training (in FAP, other psychotherapeutic modalities, or other forms of healing arts). Consultation with trusted colleagues, especially those also practicing FAP, is a critical component of both improving client care, growing as a professional, and preventing and addressing burnout.

FAP consultation teams

Sitting on a consultation team with other FAP therapists provides a truly unique context in which to learn about one's own T1s and T2s, practice courageously evoking and consequating behavior, give and receive FAP-specific case consultation, and receive support in growing as a whole person, professionally and personally. Consistent with the ideographic and contextual focus of FAP, there are no hard and fast rules that govern the operation of FAP consultation teams. Teams may be ongoing or time-limited and may be closed or open to new members; some teams may be as small as 3 members or contain as many as 15 depending on the context; teams may be facilitated consistently by

1 or 2 leaders or may rotate leadership. Team meetings typically last between 1–2 hours and occur on a weekly, bi-weekly, or monthly basis. Some teams choose to have a ritual of sharing written or video logs with each other prior to meetings related to interpersonal risks they are taking with their clients and in their outside lives and/or bridging questionnaires that function as a means of reflecting on and communicating about team processes. The format of team meetings may consist of responding to member logs (an opportunity to practice contingent responding), experiential exercises designed to evoke T1s and T2s and provide inspiration for clinical practice, as well as more traditional case consultation. Team members share their life histories and support each other in the ongoing development of a FAP therapist case conceptualization that guides both professional and personal development.

Within this one-of-a-kind setting, FAP therapists come to know one another in a profound manner. When a therapist is struggling with a clinical issue, team members are able to reflect together on how a functionally equivalent process may be occurring in the therapist's outside life or, indeed, even in the very conversation that the therapist is having with team members about the case they are presenting! The team is then well-situated to evoke a functionally equivalent improved behavior (T2) in the therapist right then and there in the context of the team meeting, and subsequently consider together how this T2 could generalize to the therapist's work with the client to address the original clinical question. For example, if a team member presents a case in which the client is consistently not completing homework assignments, the following exchange might occur:

Therapist: "It doesn't seem to matter how much we problem-solve and break the goal down into smaller and smaller pieces; the client says that they're going to do it, and then they don't."

Team Member: "How do you feel about this pattern?"
T: "I feel frustrated with myself and with the client. Under the frustration, I feel sad that we're not making more progress and then also ashamed that I'm unable to be more helpful to them."
TM: "Have you given the client any feedback about the impact of this pattern on you and your relationship with them?"

> *T:* [laughing] "No, you know I don't like giving that kind of feedback!"
>
> *TM:* "I'm aware that a number of us on the team have been late submitting our team logs or haven't submitted them at all recently. I want to invite you to take a risk: Would you please tell us candidly how it impacts you when our team falls into this pattern?"

Through this experiential practice, the therapist has the opportunity to first try out this T2 behavior (giving difficult and important feedback) within the safety of a trusted group of other mental health professionals before taking it on the road with a client. In the same way that we speak of the FAP therapy relationship as a laboratory in which clients may practice new behaviors (CRB2s) in a relatively safer and more predictable environment, both FAP consultation teams and FAP supervision constitute learning laboratories of growth for therapists where they may practice new behaviors in service of being able to skillfully implement them with clients (T2s) and in their outside lives (O2s). This form of experiential practice is especially critical in the context of learning to effectively use therapist self-disclosure as both an evoke (Rule 2) and source of reinforcement (Rule 3). To harness the power of authentic and emotionally vulnerable self-disclosure, and moreover grow the capacity to draw from this well of healing potential, therapists must be adequately acquainted with their own behavioral repertoires to ensure that they can remain sufficiently regulated to maintain awareness of their impact on the client and the client's needs as the interaction is unfolding in real time. Given the intensity and complexity of these emotionally laden exchanges with clients, as a general principle, it is advisable to first trial the strategic use of different genres of self-disclosure (e.g., features of identity, specific autobiographical memories, problematic behaviors) first with colleagues and/or supervisors prior to implementing their use with clients.

The specific topography of a FAP therapist's support infrastructure can and should shift over time and vary across individuals. What is essential is that FAP therapists (whether novices or experienced professionals) cultivate and routinely refresh their engagement with diverse resources for training, self-development, and emotional and instrumental support.

29

FAP implementation in health settings

The inherently ideographic and contextual framework of FAP makes it ideally suited for supporting clients navigating the challenging and changing stressors that accompany health-related issues. FAP is also useful for training healthcare providers in critical skills for treating emotionally distressed patients and enhancing provider-patient interactions. Given that feelings of isolation are not uncommon when encountering health-related stress, the interpersonal focus of FAP can support both patients and healthcare providers in optimizing their utilization of social support and facilitating the mutual understanding that is essential for coping with medical issues and successfully navigating demands within medical settings.

FAP for clients presenting with health-related issues

Clients may initially present for therapy due to distress related to health concerns or may already be known to the therapist when they encounter a health event. Either way, early on in the course of medical diagnosis and treatment (as well as later on whenever symptoms are acute and/or treatment demands are high), FAP sessions will typically orient more toward outside life events than under other circumstances. During these medically intensive phases, clients may be undergoing diagnostic workups, learning to manage new physical symptoms, making treatment decisions, and coping with treatment side effects, as well as adjusting to disruptions in daily functioning, relationships, long-term goals, and identity. Nevertheless, CRBs are bound to be woven throughout the client's discussion of health-related challenges. For example, consider a client who has recently received a diagnosis of metastatic cancer. When discussing their prognosis, they may become emotionally withdrawn, express dysregulated emotion, smile and talk about the importance of thinking positively, or make sarcastic jokes. Any of these behaviors could represent CRB1s, CRB2s, or neither, depending on the client's case conceptualization and the particular context of the disclosure (e.g., did the client receive new medical information two days or two months ago?).

When supporting a client in the setting of new health-related challenges, the therapist's first priority should generally be to offer attuned and non-contingent emotional and instrumental support. As the client has time to adapt to the new information (keeping in mind that the time scale of that adaptation might be weeks, months, or years), the therapist and client collaboratively have the opportunity to be curious together about the helpfulness of different strategies the client employs for responding to health-related emotional distress; it is through such conversations that CRBs relevant to the client's coping repertoire may be identified. Of particular interest from both a FAP perspective and a coping perspective, is how a client seeks and engages social support both in the setting of the therapy relationship and in outside relationships (or neglects to, as the case may be). If a therapist discovers that a client who typically feels isolated and alone in their social world has waited several sessions to disclose upsetting test results to the therapist (CRB1) or has canceled sessions in service of avoiding an opportunity to share the information, the client and therapist might collaboratively agree to begin targeting the consistent disclosure of even minor medical updates (e.g., via a routine question on the bridging questionnaire) in conjunction with homework assignments to share some of the information that is disclosed to the therapist with emotionally safe significant others during the week.

Given the intensity of emotion often elicited in association with health, disability, and mortality, therapists should be especially thoughtful regarding their use of self-disclosure in this context. While a therapist disclosing information about their own struggle with chronic illness might be profoundly validating to a client encountering a similar condition, the risk of invalidation via diverting attention from the client in a way that is misattuned (i.e., "stealing the story") and/or the client experiencing the disclosure as mismatched in emotional intensity (e.g., the client is encountering a diagnosis of metastatic cancer and the therapist, without thoughtful awareness, discloses something about their experience of coping with an early-stage cancer diagnosis) is especially high. Therefore, the consistent practice of Rule 4 (awareness of impact) is especially vital in this setting. Accessing the common humanity of suffering in the face of illness, disability, and death can be a powerful form of soothing and connection, but, as with all forms of potentially powerful reinforcement, clients will respond to it differently based on their current context and learning history. Moreover, major medical events may evoke previously extinguished patterns of both problematic and adaptive behaviors and/or introduce a new repertoire of behaviors that must be integrated into a client's evolving case conceptualization. A FAP therapy relationship ideally offers an emotionally safe setting in which to identify and practice expressing the particular emotional meanings and impacts (both painful and potentially transformative) of a health stressor such that the client can both receive effective support immediately from the therapist as well as receive guidance in generalizing the capacity to flexibly engage the social world around them as they struggle and grow in response to the shifting landscape of health adversity.

FAP groups in health settings

While one-on-one interventions are ideal for responding idiographically to clients' needs, some health settings promote group interventions. Group modalities can boost the effectiveness of interventions through the positive effects of cohesion and common humanity that emerge from a group of patients sharing common realities. This can be particularly important for patients who experience health-related stigma. FAP group modality provides a unique opportunity to help participants cultivate interpersonal skills within a safe space. These skills can be contingently reinforced by the group, along with the ability to discriminate those contextual factors that support their progress in the group, and can be tracked outside of it. The group encounter can favor a rapid generalization of skills, as it provides multiple practice opportunities and immediate consequences for them.

While FAP therapists are the main source of reinforcement for patients in individual sessions, in group settings, members are responsible for providing consequences (G-Rule 3) and presenting contextual cues that evoke patients' CRBs (G-Rule 2). Thus, group FAP therapists adopt a mediator role, engaging in two principal activities: channeling and scooping (Vandenberghe, 2016). Channeling occurs when a therapist influences the group to mobilize attention to a specific CRB emitted by one of the members. Therapists can implement four strategies for channeling: (a) Use Rule 1 to identify group dynamics that could be helpful (GRB2) or unhelpful (GRB1), (b) Use Rule 3 to provide positive reinforcement to GRB2 and differential reinforcement for GRB1, (c) Use Rules 1 and 4 to notice the effects of implementing Rule 3 on group behavior and adjust as needed, and (d) Use Rule 5 to promote the GRB2 and CRB2 out of the group. Scooping is aimed at prompting group responses to notice CRB2s from a patient when the group misses them. This can be achieved using strategies such as: (a) Using Rule 1 to notice in-session progress and group responses to CRB2s, (b) Using Rule 2 to amplify a patient's CRB2 so that the group can notice it, and (c) Using Rules 1 and 4 to track the effects of group behaviors on the patient's CRB2.

For example, we may conduct a group in a chemo room where patients gather together to receive treatment. The therapist can invite patients to share the impact that receiving the chemo is having on their lives (G-Rule 2) in order to find common humanity among the patients (GRB2) and reduce the isolationing behaviors (GRB1). Some of the expected CRB2 from patients are the common experiencing and expression of suffering, compassion, and self-compassion (maintained by social positive reinforcement), while self-invalidation, invalidation, and emotional avoidance would be conceptualized as CRB1s. To encourage patients to participate in the group, the FAP therapist can channel the group to notice the impact of the GRB1 when coming to the room and remain in silence in contrast to those moments when they sit and share their experiences (GRB2). Rule 3 can be implemented to enhance the common humanity experience in the room, and Rule 5 to create parallels on the positive effects of GRB2 when generalized beyond the group.

Implementing this group modality of FAP can greatly enhance treatment adherence in ambulatory and in-patient programs. Particularly, this modality can address one important social determinant of health: social support. FAP therapists can invite people from different programs to group sessions, where they can use group dynamics to shape interpersonal repertoires needed for strengthening their social networks, as well as developing skills to discriminate social context dynamics where such support is or is not available.

FAP in medical settings (FAP light, FAP-L)

Working with medical residents and medical students who are training in primary care and/or psychiatry offers special opportunities for introducing FAP sensitivities. These trainees, unlike people in general mental health, are typically not interested in learning FAP as a specific treatment. They are focused on work that generally is very time-limited, such as a brief appointment for a medical complaint or a medication check in psychiatry where prescribing is the main duty of the physician.

That said, there are opportunities to help physicians and other providers capture the moment in the exam room and to provide meaningful psychological connection and treatment for their patients. All physicians, while in medical school, learn to do an H&P, (a history and physical). This exam requires the physician to note and record symptoms that are occurring right here, right now. The cough right now, the belly pain right now, skin color, temperature, and so forth. The here and now focus with respect to physical symptoms can be generalized to behavioral data and can be opportunities for the physician to respond authentically and begin to shape behavior. The patient who avoids eye contact, is angry, is passive, struggles to say what is wrong, is likely providing their doctor with behavioral data with respect to how they may interact in daily life.

Helping physicians with FAP in this setting can involve helping the doctor provide in-the-moment feedback to their patients.

It is hard for me to work on helping you with your medical problem when you don't take off your dark glasses and you give terse, one-word answers to my questions… I wonder if this contributed to you being frustrated with previous doctors and why you fired them, or they fired you from their practice. I really want to help you, and I do have some ideas about how to do that. Would you be willing to take off your dark glasses while we talk so I can really see your suffering, and so you can really see my caring and attentiveness?

From the standpoint of primary care physicians, this move is consistent with their training in present moment awareness, extended to behavioral data as well as to physician private emotional responding that can guide meaningful and helpful physician-patient interactions.

Whether calling on FAP principles when treating individuals coping with serious medical illness, when facilitating support groups for patients in health settings, or when training medical providers, the flexibility of the 5 Rules can promote optimal patient coping, effective engagement in medical care, and high quality provider-patient relationships.

FAP as an integrative therapy

The scientific principles that underlie and give rise to FAP are based on learning theory and applied behavior analysis. These principles underlie all of the CBTs, though these therapies differ markedly in terms of techniques, processes, and populations of interest. Acceptance and Commitment Therapy (ACT), Dialectical Behavioral Therapy (DBT), Behavioral Activation, and other cognitive therapies share a similar backbone of looking at history, learning, and contingencies that contribute to how humans operate in the world. While Steve Hayes was in the early development of ACT, Robert Kohlenberg became aware of this, and this was one intellectual contribution to the genesis of FAP. The two therapies and developers have had deep, respectful, and mutually influential relationships with one another ever since (see Kohlenberg & Callaghan, 2010, for an account of this history).

FAP can be delivered as a stand-alone therapy and can be used alongside most any therapy to potentiate its effects. Studies have integrated FAP with Cognitive Therapy (FECT; Kohlenberg et al., 2002), ACT (FACT for smoking cessation; Gifford et al., 2011), and Behavioral Activation (FEBA for depression, Kanter et al., 2008). While each therapy system has its particular area of emphasis, FAP emphasizes the here-and-now relationship between the client and the therapist, with primacy placed on the contingencies alive between the client and the therapist as the primary vehicle of behavior change.

One of the most frequent combinations is FACT (Callaghan et al., 2004; Macías et al., 2019, Macías-Morón & Valero-Aguayo, 2021). While FAP is focused on the client's relationship with the therapist and with other people, ACT is a powerful treatment that can help people change their relationship with their own thoughts and feelings. The two inform and work beautifully together. For example:

DOI: 10.4324/9781032694832-32

C: I really didn't want to come to the session today, you pissed me off because of that thing you said about politics in the Middle East. [A CRB2, taking a risk, criticizing the therapist.]

T: I am so aware of your anger… and I am moved beyond measure that you came in to talk about it.

C: Yes, I kind of did those passengers on the bus metaphor you taught me, I had passengers telling me to blow you off, that you could never understand, that you are horrible… to cut my losses, stay home, and find a therapist more like me politically. And I know we are working on how to care even while angry and how to fight for relationships. So here I am. I didn't let the passengers drive and so here we all are, to have this uncomfortable conversation. And I still might fire you, and yet I did want to talk about it.

T: I am again beyond moved that you are trusting me with this… I know so often in the past you have run away from important relationships too fast. I want to hear more about how I angered and hurt you, while I know we don't have to agree, I am 100% sure that I respect you and your feelings and your opinions.

FACT in this way allows for a shared interweaving of the processes of defusion, in this case (i.e., loosening the practice of seeing one's thoughts as completely true assessments of the world), and FAP's emphasis on how one's manner of relating to those thoughts might be impacting the quality of the client's relationships or the degree of connection or isolation they are feeling in the world. Put more simply, both ACT and FAP, like other contextual behavior therapies, encourage a client to orient their attention more to their context and the outer world, rather than an inner world filled with the certainty of thoughts that arise in the echo chamber of our own mind.

Training in ACT can also be helpful and improve the skills of a FAP therapist, as moving between the five rules relies heavily upon a therapist and client's ability in perspective-taking, a shared therapeutic target. An ACT therapist might encourage a client to consider experiencing the self through the eyes of another ("how do you think she saw you?"), the self across time ("how will you feel about this decision looking back from the end of life?"), or across physical space ("what would you think watching yourself do this from across the street?"), all grounded in a behavioral model of language that underlies ACT, relational frame theory. In FAP, we use a similar strategy in in-to-out or out-to-in reflections (see Chapter 24 on Rule 5) that rely on broadening a client's capacity to consider how we might see, value, and care for them, or how they might feel compassion toward themselves during difficult past or future moments or times in their life.

Fear of love, fear of loving

Another powerful, related approach that we have found valuable in integrating into FAP work is Compassion-Focused Therapy (CFT; Gilbert, 2010). CFT draws on evolution, affective neuroscience, and cognitive behavior therapy techniques to consider how a lack of social safety drives shame, self-criticism, and the maintenance or recurrence of psychological distress across a variety of diagnoses. CFT considers the difficulties that arise from a fear of receiving love or compassion from others (e.g., it will be too painful when they fail me), to give compassion to others (e.g., I will be used or treated like a sucker for giving too much), or to give compassion to the self (e.g., if I stop criticizing myself, how will I ever improve?). Techniques such as meditation, visualization, or other practices might be used to challenge those fears or expand one's capacity to feel or experience the interoceptive sensations of giving or receiving compassion without becoming overwhelmed.

While FAP and CFT share a belief in the importance of close and meaningful relationships in one's life, and center relationships as key to thriving, the emphasis differs. Most CFT practices emphasize individual exercise or practice outside of the room, and while it is implicit in the approach that the therapist should be a compassionate person, there is less guidance on how the therapeutic relationship might be used as a tool to foster or promote self-compassion. FAP, on the other hand, centers on the direct, lived experience of mutually exchanging feelings of warmth and care in the present moment. It is the therapeutic encounter in which a client might most vividly be challenged to receive warmth from another or to try out giving it to either the therapist or themselves. As clinicians with experience training from CFT teachers, there is also the invaluable insight offered in many CFT models that for those who have experienced profound mistreatment, neglect, or betrayal in the development of early life relationships, this history may result in too much warmth being experienced as punishing or aversive. This is an important consideration for the FAP therapist who, in addition to Rule 4, should be ready to gradually expose a client to experiencing warmth in the room, rather than overwhelming or punishing a client with it from the start.

References

American Psychiatric Association. (2000). *Diagnostic and statistical manual of mental disorders: DSM-IV-TR*. Washington, DC: American Psychiatric Association.

Barrett, M. D., & Berman, J. S. (2001). Is psychotherapy more effective when therapists disclose information about themselves? *Journal of Consulting and Clinical Psychology, 69*, 597–603.

Baruch, D. E., Kanter, J. W., Busch, A. B., & Juskiewicz, K. (2009a). Enhancing the therapy relationship in acceptance and commitment therapy for psychotic symptoms. *Clinical Case Studies, 8*, 241–257. https://doi.org/10.1177/1534650109334818

Beck, A. T., Rush, A. J., Shaw, B. F., & Emery, G. (1979). *The cognitive therapy of depression*. New York: Guilford Press.

Bolling, M. Y., Terry, C. M., & Kohlenberg, R. (2006). Behavioral theories. In *Comprehensive handbook of personality and psychopathology, vol. 1: Personality and everyday functioning* (pp. 142–157). Hoboken, NJ: John Wiley & Sons Inc.

Bowen, S., Haworth, K., Grow, J., Tsai, M., & Kohlenberg R. J. (2012). Interpersonal mindfulness informed by functional analytic psychotherapy: Findings from a pilot randomized trial. *International Journal of Behavioral Consultation and Therapy, 7*(2), 125–134. https://doi.org/10.1037/h0100931

Callaghan, G. M. (2006a). The Functional Idiographic Assessment Template (FIAT) System: For use with interpersonally-based interventions including Functional Analytic Psychotherapy (FAP) and FAP-enhanced treatments. *The Behavior Analyst Today, 7*, 357–398. https://doi.org/10.1037/h0100160

Callaghan, G. M. (2006b). Functional analytic psychotherapy and supervision. *International Journal of Behavioral and Consultation Therapy, 2*, 416–431. https://doi.org/10.1037/h0100794

Callaghan, G. M., Gregg, J. A., Marx, B., Kohlenberg, B. S., & Gifford, E. (2004). FACT: The utility of an integration of Functional Analytic Psychotherapy and Acceptance and Commitment Therapy to alleviate human suffering. *Psychotherapy: Theory, Research, Practice, Training, 41*, 195–207. https://doi.org/10.1037/0033-3204.41.3.195

Chambless, D. L., & Hollon, S. D. (1998). Defining empirically supported therapies. *Journal of Consulting and Clinical Psychology, 66*(1), 7–18. https://doi.org/10.1037/0022-006X.66.1.7

Clark, D. A., Beck, A. T., & Alford, B. A. (1999). *Scientific foundations of cognitive theory and therapy of depression.* New York: John Wiley and Sons, Inc.

Cooper, J. O., Heron, T. E., & Heward, W. L. (2020). *Applied behavior analysis* (3rd ed.). Pearson.

Cordova, J. V., & Scott, R. L. (2001). Intimacy: A behavioral interpretation. *Behavior Analyst, 24*(1), 75–86. https://doi.org/10.1007/BF03392020

Cuthbert, B. N., & Insel, T. R. (2013). Toward the future of psychiatric diagnosis: The seven pillars of RDoC. *BMC Medicine, 11,* 126–134. https://doi.org/10.1186/1741-7015-11-126

Darrow, S. M., Callaghan, G. M., Bonow, J. T., & Follette, W. C. (2014). The functional idiographic assessment template-questionnaire (FIAT-Q): Initial psychometric properties. *Journal of Contextual Behavioral Science, 3*(2), 124–135. https://doi.org/10.1016/j.jcbs.2014.02.002

Deikman, A. J. (1973). The meaning of everything. In R. E. Ornstein (Ed.), *The nature of human consciousness.* San Francisco: Freeman.

Edwards, C. E., & Murdock, N. L. (1994). Characteristics of therapist self-disclosure in the counseling process. *Journal of Counseling and Development, 72,* 384–389. https://doi.org/10.1002/j.1556-6676.1994.tb00954.x

Erikson, E. (1968). *Identity, youth, and crisis.* New York: Norton.

Ethical Principles of Psychologists and Code of Conduct, 2010 Amendments. (2010). Retrieved January 2, 2011, from http://www.apa.org/ethics/code/index.aspx

Ferster, C. B. (1967a). The transition from laboratory to clinic. *The Psychological Record, 17,* 145–150.

Ferster, C. B. (1967b). Arbitrary and natural reinforcement. *The Psychological Record, 17,* 341–347.

Ferster, C. B. (1979). A laboratory model of psychotherapy: The boundary between clinical practice and experimental psychology. *Trends in Behavior Therapy,* 23–38.

Follette, W. C., & Callaghan, G. M. (1995). Do as I do, not as I say: A behavior-analytic approach to supervision. *Professional Psychology: Research & Practice, 26,* 413–421. https://doi.org/10.1037/0735-7028.26.4.413

Follette, W. C., Naugle, A. E., & Callaghan, G. M. (1996). A radical behavioral understanding of the therapeutic relationship in effecting change. *Behavior Therapy, 27*(4), 623–641. https://doi.org/10.1016/S0005-7894(96)80047-5

Follette, W. C., Naugle, A. E., & Linnerooth, P. J. (2000). Functional alternatives to traditional assessment and diagnosis. In M. Dougher (Ed.), *Clinical behavior analysis.* Context Press, Reno.

Gifford, E. V., Kohlenberg, B. S., Hayes, S. C., Pierson, H. M., Piasecki, M. P., Antonuccio, D. O., & Palm, K. M. (2011). Does acceptance and relationship focused behavior therapy contribute to bupropion outcomes? A randomized controlled trial of functional analytic psychotherapy and acceptance and commitment therapy for smoking cessation. *Behavior Therapy, 42*(4), 700–715. https://doi.org/10.1016/j.beth.2011.03.002

Gilbert, P. (2010). *Compassion focused therapy: Distinctive features.* Routledge.

Hanley, G. P., Iwata, B. A., & McCord, B. E. (2003). Functional analysis of problem behavior: A review. *Journal of Applied Behavior Analysis, 36*(2), 147–185.

Hardebeck, E. J. (2023). Living with awareness, courage, and love: An accessible behavioral intervention to improve well-being [Doctoral dissertation, Antioch University]. OhioLINK ETD Center. http://rave.ohiolink.edu/etdc /view?acc_num=antioch1682364123339956

Haworth, K., Kanter, J., Tsai, M., Kuczynski, A., Rae, J., & Kohlenberg, R. J. (2015). Reinforcement matters: A preliminary, laboratory-based component-process analysis of functional analytic psychotherapy's model of social connection. *Journal of Contextual Behavioral Science, 4*(4), 281–291. https://doi.org/10.1016/j.jcbs.2015.08.003

Hayes, S. C. (1984). Making sense of spirituality. *Behaviorism, 12*(2), 99–110.

Hayes, S. C., Barnes Holmes, D., & Roche, B. (Eds.). (2001). *Relational frame theory: A post-Skinnerian account of human language and cognition.* New York, NY: Kluwer Academic/Plenum Publishers; Springer Science & Business Media.

Hayes, S. C., & Brownstein, A. J. (1986). Mentalism, behavior-behavior relations, and a behavior-analytic view of the purposes of science. *Behavior Analyst, 9*(2), 175–190. https://doi.org/10.1007/BF03391944

Hayes, S. C., Hofmann, S. G., & Ciarrochi, J. (2020). A process-based approach to psychological diagnosis and treatment: The conceptual and treatment utility of an extended evolutionary meta model. *Clinical Psychology Review, 82*, 101908. https://doi.org/10.1016/j.cpr.2020.101908

Hayes, S. C., Strosahl, K. D., & Wilson, K. G. (1999). *Acceptance and commitment therapy: An experiential approach to behavior change.* New York: Guilford Press.

Hayes, S. C., & Toarmino, D. (1995). If behavioral principles are generally applicable, why is it necessary to understand cultural diversity? *the Behavior Therapist, 18*, 21–23.

Hill, C. E., Helms, J. E., Tichenor, V., Spiegel, S. B., O'Grady, K. E., & Perry, E. S. (1988). The effects of therapist response modes in brief psychotherapy. *Journal of Counseling Psychology, 35*, 222–233. https://doi.org/10.1037 /10412-004

Hineline, P. N. (1983). When we speak of knowing. *The Behavior Analyst, 6*(2), 183–186. https://doi.org/10.1007/BF03392398

Hofmann, S. G., & Hayes, S. C. (2019). The future of intervention science: Process-based therapy. *Clinical Psychological Science, 7*(1), 37–50. https://doi.org/10.1177/2167702618772296

Holman, G., Kohlenberg, R. J., & Tsai, M. (2012). Development and preliminary evaluation of a FAP protocol: Brief relationship enhancement. *International Journal of Behavioral Consultation and Therapy, 7*(2), 52–57. https://doi.org/10.1037/h0100937

Horvath, A. O. (2001). The alliance. *Psychotherapy, 38*(4), 365–372. https://doi.org/10.1037/0033-3204.38.4.365

Kanter, J. W., Kohlenberg, R. J., & Loftus, E. F. (2004). Experimental and psychotherapeutic demand characteristics and the cognitive therapy rationale: An analogue study. *Cognitive Therapy and Research, 28*(2), 229–239.

Kanter, J. W., Kuczynski, A., Tsai, M., & Kohlenberg, R. J. (2018). A brief contextual behavioral intervention to improve relationships: A randomized trial. *Journal of Contextual Behavioral Science, 10,* 75–84. https://doi.org/10.1016/j.jcbs.2018.09.001

Kanter, J. W., Landes, S. J., Busch, A. M., Rusch, L. C., Brown, K. R., Baruch, D. E., & Holman, G. (2006). The effect of contingent reinforcement on target variables in outpatient psychotherapy for depression: A successful and unsuccessful case using functional analytic psychotherapy. *Journal of Applied Behavior Analysis, 39,* 463–467.

Kanter, J. W., Manbeck, K. E., Kuczynski, A. M., Maitland, D. W. M., Villas-Bôas, A., & Reyes Ortega, M. A. (2017). A comprehensive review of research on Functional Analytic Psychotherapy. *Clinical Psychology Review, 58,* 141–156.

Kanter, J. W., Manos, R. C., Busch, A. M., & Rusch, L. C. (2008). Making behavioral activation more behavioral. *Behavior Modification, 32*(6), 780–803. https://doi.org/10.1177/0145445508317265

Kanter, J., Tsai, M., & Kohlenberg, R. J. (Eds.). (2010). *The practice of functional analytic psychotherapy.* New York: Springer.

Knox, S., & Hill, C. E. (2003). Therapist self-disclosure: Research based suggestions for practitioners. *Journal of Clinical Psychology/In Session, 59,* 529–539. https://doi.org/10.1002/jclp.10157

Kohlenberg, B. S., & Callaghan, G. M. (2010). FAP and acceptance commitment therapy (ACT): Similarities, divergence, and integration. In J. W. Kanter, M. Tsai, & R. J. Kohlenberg (Eds.), *The practice of functional analytic psychotherapy* (pp. 31–46). New York: Springer.

Kohlenberg, R. J., & Tsai, M. (1991). *Functional analytic psychotherapy: Creating intense and curative therapeutic relationships.* New York: Plenum Press.

Kohlenberg, R. J., Kanter, J. W., Bolling, M. Y., Parker, C., & Tsai, M. (2002). Enhancing cognitive therapy for depression with functional analytic psychotherapy: Treatment guidelines and empirical findings. *Cognitive and Behavioral Practice, 9*(3), 213–229.

Kohlenberg, R. J., Kanter, J. W., Tsai, M., & Weeks, C. E. (2010). FAP and cognitive behavior therapy. In J. W. Kanter, M. Tsai, & R. J. Kohlenberg (Eds.), *The practice of functional analytic psychotherapy* (pp. 11–30). New York: Springer.

Kohlenberg, R. J., Tsai, M., Kanter, J. W., & Parker, C. R. (2009). Self and mindfulness. In M. Tsai, R. J. Kohlenberg, J. W. Kanter, B. Kohlenberg, W. C. Follette, & G. M. Callaghan (Eds.), *A guide to functional analytic psychotherapy: Awareness, courage, love and behaviorism* (pp. 103–130). New York: Springer.

Kohlenberg, R. J., Tsai, M., Kuczynski, A. M., Rae, J. R., Lagbas, E., Lo, J., & Kanter, J. W. (2015). A brief, interpersonally oriented mindfulness intervention incorporating Functional Analytic Psychotherapy's model of awareness, courage and love. *Journal of Contextual Behavioral Science, 4*(2), 107–111. https://doi.org/10.1016/j.jcbs.2015.03.003

Kohut, H. (1971). *The analysis of the self.* New York: International Universities Press.

Kuei, T., Tsai, M., McLeod, H., White, R., & Kanter, J. (2018). Using the Primary Process Emotional-Behavioural System (PPEB) to better meet patient needs in psychotherapy. *Clinical Psychology & Psychotherapy, 26*(1), 55–73. https://doi.org/10.1002/cpp.2330

Longmore, R. J., & Worrell, M. (2007). Do we need to challenge thoughts in cognitive behavior therapy? *Clinical Psychology Review, 27*(2), 173–187.

Macías, J., Valero-Aguayo, L., Bond, F. W., & Blanca, M. J. (2019). The efficacy of functional-analytic psychotherapy and acceptance and commitment therapy (FACT) for public employees. *Psicothema, 31*(1), 24–29. https://doi.org/10.7334/psicothema2018.202z

Maitland, D., Hardebeck, E., Pedersen, K., Moore, E., Wahl, L., & Tsai, M. (2024). Using functional analytic psychotherapy's awareness, courage, and love model to generate open-heartedness towards others: A pilot randomized controlled trial. Manuscript submitted for publication.

Maitland, D. W. M. (2024). The extended evolutionary meta-model and process-based therapy: Contemporary lenses for understanding functional analytic psychotherapy. *Journal of Contextual Behavioral Science, 32*, 100750. https://doi.org/10.1016/j.jcbs.2024.100750

Martell, C. R., Dimidjian, S., & Herman-Dunn, R. (2010). *Behavioral activation for depression: A clinician's guide.* New York: Guilford.

Masterson, J. F. (1985). *The real self.* New York: Brunner/Mazel.

McIlvane, W. (2013). Simple and complex discrimination learning. In G. Madden (Ed.), *APA handbook of behavior analysis* (Vol. 2). American Psychology Association.

Miller, A., Williams, M. T., Wetterneck, C. T., Kanter, J., & Tsai, M. (2015). Using functional analytic psychotherapy to improve awareness and connection in racially diverse client-therapist dyads. *The Behavior Therapist, 38*(6), 150–156.

Montoya-Rodríguez, M. M., Molina, F. J., & McHugh, L. (2017). A review of relational frame theory research into deictic relational responding. *The Psychological Record, 67,* 569–579. https://doi.org/10.1007/s40732-016-0216-x

Macías-Morón, J. J. M., & Valero-Aguayo, L. (2021). Applications of FACT in the academic context to improve the health of high school students. *Psicología Conductual, 29*(3), 579–595. https://doi.org/10.51668/bp.8321304n

Milne, D., & James, I. (2000). A systematic review of effective cognitive-behavioural supervision. *British Journal of Clinical Psychology, 39*(2), 111–127.

Muñoz-Martínez, A. M., & Follette, W. C. (2019). When love is not enough: The case of therapeutic love as a middle-level term in functional analytic psychotherapy. Behavior Analysis: Research and Practice, 19(1), 103–113. https://doi.org/10.1037/bar0000141

Muñoz-Martínez, A. M., Stanton, C. E., Ta, J. D., Molaie, A. M., & Follette, W. C. (2022). Linking process to outcome in Functional Analytic Psychotherapy: Evaluating the behavioral mechanism of change of a process-based therapy. *Journal of Contextual Behavioral Science, 24,* 102–111. https://doi.org/10.1016/j.jcbs.2022.04.001

Nelson, K. M., Yang, J. P., Maliken, A. C., Tsai, M., & Kohlenberg, R. J. (2016). Introduction to using structured evocative activities in functional analytic psychotherapy. *Cognitive and Behavioral Practice, 23*(4), 459–463. https://doi.org/10.1016/j.cbpra.2013.12.009

Neville, H. A., Awad, G. H., Brooks, J. E., Flores, M. P., & Bluemel, J. (2013). Color-blind racial ideology: Theory, training, and measurement implications in psychology. *American Psychologist, 68*(6), 455–466.

Nichols, M. P., & Efran, J. (1985). Catharsis in psychotherapy: A new perspective. *Psychotherapy: Theory, Research and Practice, 22*(1), 46–58. https://doi.org/10.1037/h0088525

Pedersen, K., Stidhams, S., & Tsai, M. (2024). A brief behavioral intervention to increase social connection in college students: A randomized controlled trial. Manuscript submitted for publication.

Rogers, C. R. (1961). *On becoming a person.* Boston: Houghton Mifflin.

Safran, J. D., & Muran, J. C. (2001). A relational approach to training and supervision in cognitive psychotherapy. *Journal of Cognitive Psychotherapy, 15,* 3–15.

Sanford, B. T., Ciarrochi, J., Hofmann, S. G., Chin, F., Gates, K. M., & Hayes, S. C. (2022). Toward empirical process-based case conceptualization: An idionomic network examination of the process-based assessment tool. *Journal of Contextual Behavioral Science, 25*, 10–25. https://doi.org/10.1016/j.jcbs.2022.05.006

Shapiro, J. L. (1987). Message from the masters on breaking old ground? The Evolution of Psychotherapy Conference. *Psychotherapy in Private Practice, 5*(3), 65–72.

Sinclair, S., Raffin-Bouchal, S., Venturato, L., Mijovic-Kondejewski, J., & Smith-MacDonald, L. (2017). Compassion fatigue: A meta-narrative review of the healthcare literature. *International Journal of Nursing Studies, 69*, 9–24.

Singh, R. S., & O'Brien, W. H. (2018). A quantitative synthesis of functional analytic psychotherapy single-subject research. *Journal of Contextual Behavioral Science, 7*, 35–46. https://doi.org/10.1016/j.jcbs.2017.11.004

Skinner, B. F. (1957). *Verbal behavior.* East Norwalk, CT: Appleton-Century-Crofts.

Skinner, B. F. (1974). *About behaviorism.* New York: Knopf.

Spitzberg, B. H., & Cupach, W. R. (1989). *Handbook of interpersonal competence research.* New York: Springer Science & Business Media.

Stokes, T. F., & Baer, D. M. (1977). An implicit technology of generalization 1. *Journal of Applied Behavior Analysis, 10*(2), 349–367.

Tolin, D. F., McKay, D., Forman, E. M., Klonsky, E. D., & Thombs, B. D. (2015). Empirically supported treatment: Recommendations for a new model. *Clinical Psychology: Science and Practice, 22*(4), 317–338. https://doi.org/10.1037/h0101729

Törneke, N., Luciano, C., & Salas, S. V. (2008). Rule-governed behavior and psychological problems. *International Journal of Psychology and Psychological Therapy, 8*(2), 141–156.

Tsai, M., Callaghan, G. M., & Kohlenberg, R. J. (2013). The use of awareness, courage, therapeutic love, and behavioral interpretation in functional analytic psychotherapy. *Psychotherapy, 50*(3), 366.

Tsai, M., Callaghan, G. M., Kohlenberg, R. J., Follette, W. C., & Darrow, S. M. (2009). Supervision and therapist self-development. In M. Tsai, R. J. Kohlenberg, J. W. Kanter, B. Kohlenberg, W. C. Follette, & G. M. Callaghan (Eds.), *A guide to functional analytic psychotherapy: Awareness, courage, love and behaviorism* (pp. 167–198). New York: Springer.

Tsai, M., Gustafsson, T., Kanter, J., Plummer Loudon, M., & Kohlenberg, R. J. (2017). Saying good goodbyes to your clients: A functional analytic psychotherapy (FAP) perspective. *Psychotherapy, 54*(1), 22–28. https://doi.org/10.1037/pst0000091

Tsai, M., Hardebeck, E., Ramos, F., Turlove, H., Nordal-Jonsson, K., Vongdala, A., Zhang, W., & Kohlenberg, R. J. (2020). Helping couples connect during the COVID-19 pandemic: A pilot randomised controlled trial of an awareness, courage, and love intervention. *Applied Psychology Health and Well-being, 12*(4), 1140–1156. https://doi.org/10.1111/aphw.12241

Tsai, M., Mandell, T., Maitland, D., Kanter, J., & Kohlenberg, R. J. (2016). Reducing inadvertent clinical errors: Guidelines from functional analytic psychotherapy. *Psychotherapy, 53*(3), 331–335. https://doi.org/10.1037/pst0000065

Tsai, M., McKelvie, M., Kohlenberg, R., & Kanter, J. (2014). Functional analytic psychotherapy: Using awareness, courage and love in treatment. Society for the Advancement of Psychotherapy. http://societyforpsychotherapy.org/functional-analytic-psychotherapy-fap-using-awareness-courage-love-treatment/

Tsai, M., Plummer, M., Kanter, J., Newring, R., & Kohlenberg, R. (2010). Therapist grief and functional analytic psychotherapy: Strategic self-disclosure of personal loss. *Journal of Contemporary Psychotherapy, 40*(1), 1–10.

Tsai, M., Yoo, D., Hardebeck, E., Plummer Loudon, M., & Kohlenberg, R. J. (2019). Creating safe, evocative, attuned, and mutually vulnerable therapeutic beginnings: Strategies from functional analytic psychotherapy. *Psychotherapy, 56*(1), 55–61. https://doi.org/10.1037/pst0000203.

Vandenberghe, L. (2016). A logical framework for functional analytic group therapy. *Cognitive and Behavioral Practice, 23*(4), 464–472. https://doi.org/10.1016/j.cbpra.2015.09.005

Watkins, C. E., Jr. (1990). The effects of counselor self-disclosure: A research review. *The Counseling Psychologist, 18*, 477–500. https://doi.org/10.1177/0011000090183009

Williams, B. A. (1983). Revising the principle of reinforcement. *Behaviorism, 11*(1), 63–88.

Index

Printed in the United States
by Baker & Taylor Publisher Services